I0693366

Uncertain Grace

One Couple's Journey Through Cancer

Dr. Melanie Dunlap

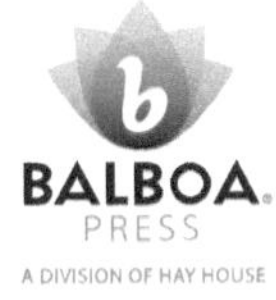

BALBOA.
PRESS

A DIVISION OF HAY HOUSE

Balboa Press books may be ordered through booksellers or by contacting:

Balboa Press
A Division of Hay House
1663 Liberty Drive
Bloomington, IN 47403
www.balboapress.com
1 (877) 407-4847

Because of the dynamic nature of the Internet, any web addresses or links contained in this book may have changed since publication and may no longer be valid. The views expressed in this work are solely those of the author and do not necessarily reflect the views of the publisher, and the publisher hereby disclaims any responsibility for them.

This book is a work of non-fiction. Unless otherwise noted, the author and the publisher make no explicit guarantees as to the accuracy of the information contained in this book and in some cases, names of people and places have been altered to protect their privacy.

The author of this book does not dispense medical advice or prescribe the use of any technique as a form of treatment for physical, emotional, or medical problems without the advice of a physician, either directly or indirectly. The intent of the author is only to offer information of a general nature to help you in your quest for emotional and spiritual well-being. In the event you use any of the information in this book for yourself, which is your constitutional right, the author and the publisher assume no responsibility for your actions.

Any people depicted in stock imagery provided by Getty Images are models, and such images are being used for illustrative purposes only. Certain stock imagery © Getty Images.

Print information available on the last page.

ISBN: 978-1-9822-1212-4 (sc)
ISBN: 978-1-9822-1214-8 (hc)
ISBN: 978-1-9822-1213-1 (e)

Library of Congress Control Number: 2018910857

Balboa Press rev. date: 09/17/2018

DEDICATION

This book is dedicated to my loving husband Tom, my soulmate, my partner, my one true love.

CONTENTS

ACKNOWLEDGEMENTS

A special thank you to Lisa Vallee for always providing the right balance of love and comfort.

Thank you to the women in my circle who cried with me, laughed with me, and held me during the most difficult times.

Thank you to the entire Peaceful Spirit Enrichment Center community for their outpouring of love, support, and generosity during this journey.

Thank you to my coach and editor, Charles Grosel of Write for Success, for helping me turn a series of blogs into this book.

PREFACE

It was a simple herbal workshop that started my journey into natural health. I became a master herbalist, got into energy work, massage therapy, and a few other modalities, and eventually worked my way to a Doctor of Naturopathy degree. I've always felt the call to be a healer.

I am very good at taking care of other people. I am not as good about taking care of myself, but I am getting better at it every day. This past year and a half put both of these to the test, as my husband, Tom, and I were both treated for cancer—mine, breast cancer, and his, lung cancer. *How can this happen?* I yelled at the universe time and time again. It wasn't supposed to be this way.

And yet there it was. These tirades did not faze the universe in the least, and I had to get down to the job of working to heal myself and Tom. It was a grueling, tearful, heartrending, and trying time for both of us, physically and emotionally. We each had to face our own pain and mortality head on, and then the universe, that jokester, doubled down and forced us to face the pain and mortality of the love of our life, our soul mate, the one who each of us would have given anything to save from that experience. And though it's not quite over—it never is quite over where cancer is concerned—we made it through with fear, hard work, love, anger, grit, joy, sadness, help from our friends and family, and a flood of tears.

Through it all, I kept a blog on my web site, MelanieDunlap. com. I write blogs regularly for the site on all kinds of topics related to natural health, including self-care, stress, inflammation, and poop.

Yes, I wrote a blog about poop. The state of your poop has a lot to do with your health. Check it out.

So it only seemed natural when I found myself challenged by cancer that I would blog about the experience. I did so for many reasons. To keep track of the experience while I was in the middle of it so I wouldn't forget the details. To meditate on my state of mind and feelings. To stay centered. To vent. To keep friends and family informed. To show others undergoing similar challenges a path through (not *the* path, but *a* path). And to keep things as normal as possible during this huge disruption in our lives.

Many of our friends and loved ones who supported us in person and by following the blog have told me, "You've got to get this out there. You've got to write a book. It will help so many people."

They had me at "help so many people." After all, that's my job. That's my calling. And though I knew it wouldn't be easy to revisit this journey, I know it's worth it if I can help at least one reader walk this path with less fear and a few useful tools.

So here it is—the story of our journey through cancer, and the uncertain grace with which we have been blessed.

INTRODUCTION

But first, a little more about Tom and me.

As I mentioned in the Preface, I have a degree as a naturopathic doctor, but I don't work in the conventional manner. I have a wide skillset. I am an herbalist, wellness educator and coach, a sound and energy healer, a Labyrinth facilitator, a Reiki master, and a massage therapist. Oh, and a business owner. Helping people find their own unique path to personal wellness is my passion and my vocation. I blend and sell hand-made herbal and natural remedies through Aunt Mel's Herbs & Insights, and I give workshops on healing and wellness, host healing ceremonies and spiritual events, including our well-known Full Moon Labyrinth Walks, and coach clients at the Peaceful Spirit Enrichment Center, which I founded in 2008.

I'm not telling you all of this to blow my own horn, but to let you know where I'm coming from.

The Peaceful Spirit Enrichment Center is set in the desert foothills of New River, Arizona, among giant Saguaros and Palo Verde and Ironwood trees. On any given day, we see wild rabbits, quail, and roadrunners on the grounds, while hawks circle intently above. At night we hear the howling of coyotes, the rustle of foxes, the hooting of owls. We have our own chickens for fresh eggs. Our neighbors have horses, goats, and ATVs, and almost everyone drives a pick-up or SUV. Part Wild West, part spiritual retreat, all ours. (Well, ours and the bank's if you want to be technical.) We're far enough from metropolitan Phoenix for peace and solitude, yet close enough—as you will soon learn—to drive into town for, say, medical treatments.

The Center is sacred ground for Tom and me, where our lifelong quest for health and enlightenment comes together. Here I can help clients achieve balance of body, mind, and spirit, and sometimes I can even achieve this balance for myself. The Center has a Labyrinth to tap into the healing powers of the Earth, meditation gardens, a fairy village, statues of the Lady and the Buddha, a prayer tree, and a retreat space called Sunshine House. The Center is my place of business and my refuge. I am renewed when I spend time with the beautiful plants and herbs, tend the fairy garden, walk the Labyrinth, and hang out with family and friends. My cup runs over with gratitude and love each and every day.

I always knew I wanted to help people heal, and in another life I might have become a medical doctor. I didn't really have the education for that in this life, however, nor the financial means, and I began in the healing profession as a phlebotomist on the psychiatric floor of a hospital. This was a stressful and sometimes dangerous job—not all of the patients wanted their blood taken—so I began looking for a different job in the healing professions and ended up almost by chance taking classes to become an herbalist. I say by chance because the herbal classes were the classes being offered at the time I enrolled at the North Carolina School of Natural Healing, so an herbalist I became. When we moved to Arizona, I did something I vowed I would never do—became a massage therapist and added these skills to my healing toolbox. Meanwhile, I started my studies in naturopathy, and in June of 2017, I received my degree.

I couldn't run the Peaceful Spirit Enrichment Center without Tom. His title on the Center's website is Facilities Director and Resident Artist, but Tom is so much more than that. He is my husband, my lover, and my best friend. He has the strength and stamina of the biker, trucker, and mechanic he has been for most of his life and the heart and vision of an artist, which he has been for even more of his life. Tom keeps me grounded and the Center humming. He's the one who designed and maintains the Labyrinth, and he's the one who takes care of the grounds and sets up for our events. He puts up the tents and canopies, arranges the chairs, splits wood for the fire pits, rakes the paths—and then tears it all down afterwards. If a chair breaks or a table wobbles, he'll fix it. If light bulbs burn out, he'll replace them. If a tree blows over in the wind—well, he'll clear it out of the path, if necessary, but otherwise he'll leave it where it fell. He has the eye of an artist, and the found art of nature is profoundly beautiful to him.

Which may be why he expresses his art mostly in wood, as a self-taught pyrographer—that's wood burner for us lay people. His beautiful artwork is displayed throughout the Center—hand-turned wooden bowls; wood-burned pieces on spiritual and mystical themes, such as signs of the zodiac, wizards, wise women, the Lady of the Lake; and carvings of natural and mystical creatures from humpbacked whales to dragons. He burned a series of antique firetrucks that are hanging in the Hall of Flame Museum in Phoenix—yes, we both see the irony. I am happy and proud to say that Tom is a full-time artist now, his duties at the Center notwithstanding.

The point is, we had both come to very good places in our lives. Despite the usual ups and downs of business owners—the not-so-well attended event, the windstorm the afternoon of a full moon walk, a faulty septic system—both of us were living our dreams, and life was just so damn good.

We never saw it coming.

CHAPTER 1

If you've read this far, you've figured out that I am anything but conventional. Just so I didn't get too predictable in my unconventionality, however, at the advice of my doctor, I decided to follow the conventional path and get a mammogram. Plus, my insurance would pay for it. Like so many others, many of my medical decisions are based on what the insurance company is willing to cover. This was early in June 2016.

I'm not a fan of mammograms—I don't care what people tell you, they hurt!—but for Western medical technology, they are the conventional means of detecting breast cancer. Not perfect by any means, but fairly effective. Not that I had anything to worry about. This was going to be strictly routine.

I was convinced I didn't really need the mammogram, and I almost cancelled the appointment at the last minute. But I had already scheduled the procedure, and I usually do what I say I'm going to do. I hauled my happy self to the breast health center, though reluctantly. It was early in the morning, and there was no reason to drag anyone else into this.

As these things go, the procedure went quickly. The paperwork, the instructions, the robe, a brief wait, the tear-inducing crushing of the breasts, the buzz of the machine, the getting dressed, the neutral, "Have a good day, you'll get a call in a few days." I was in and out without a fuss, glad it was over.

Except—it wasn't over.

Less than 48 hours later I got a call from the doctor's office. They had seen something on the mammogram and wanted to investigate further. I needed to come in for an ultrasound on my right breast. "O-kay," I said. We scheduled the appointment for five days later.

I wouldn't say I worried every second of those days leading up to the next appointment, but whenever my mind wandered, it definitely made its way to that subject. But I had been called back before for a follow-up ultrasound, and those had worked out fine. Nothing to it. I'd go back, get a clean bill of health, get on with my life. I didn't make a big deal about it. I didn't meditate on it. I didn't ask my inner healer what she thought. I didn't even tell anyone but Tom about the second appointment. I just let it be and tried not to overthink it.

Loving man that he is, Tom offered to go with me this time, but I said no, I wanted to go alone. I justified that decision by telling myself things like, his back hurts if he sits too long; he won't be comfortable just waiting; he has more important things to do, like his art or something for the Center. These were much better uses of his time, I convinced myself.

What I was really doing was letting my own self-esteem issues get in the way, issues left over from an abusive childhood I'm not going to go into great detail about. I'm also a country girl from the South, strong and independent. I don't want to inconvenience anyone. I don't deserve—or even want—any, let alone extra, attention. I take care of others, they don't take care of me. Besides, if I asked Tom to go, I'd be admitting it was serious. And it wasn't. Serious. Was it?

It wasn't serious. Until it was. When I stepped through the office doors, it hit me. I felt nervous. Even though I hadn't sat in dialogue with my inner healer, she had been whispering in my ear, vying for attention. She had something important to say, and finally she got through to me—this wouldn't be an all-clear.

I pushed that thought away, checked in, and sat down to wait. I picked up a magazine off the table to pass the time, then dropped it in irritation. I couldn't make out any words but the headlines without reading glasses, and I didn't feel like digging through my bag to get them. I drummed my fingers, tried some breathing exercises.

Fortunately, it was just a short time in the lobby before they called my name.

As I followed the nurse through the door, I could feel myself shaking. I took a deep breath and tried to pay attention to what she was saying. Put on this robe, store your stuff in the locker, and take the key with you. Got it.

At least the robes were much better than the old paper gowns they used to give you for these kinds of examinations.

I took a seat in the inner waiting room with several other women, all wearing the same style robes. It reminded me of the time I had gone to a fancy spa, and we all sat around in bulky, soft robes drinking juice and waiting for our massages. We were relaxed and chatty, looking forward to a little Me time. No one in this room was relaxed or chatty or looking forward to her appointment. We all had a version of the deer-in-the-headlights look.

When the technician came to get me, she confirmed that I was scheduled to have an ultrasound on my right breast. But then she surprised me by saying they also wanted to do another mammogram on my left breast to clarify something they had seen there.

Wait. No. I wasn't ready for both my breasts to be under scrutiny. My anxiety level went up a notch. Double the procedures, double the anxiety—or more.

I felt very vulnerable lying on the ultrasound table with one breast exposed, tightly covering my other one with the robe as if somehow I could protect it. I'll admit as a naturopath I'm not a fan of the medical machine that is healthcare in the United States, but the women who worked with me that day were caring, compassionate, and very professional.

The tech's tone was comforting as she explained how the ultrasound would go. She needed to see if she could locate what they had found suspicious on the mammogram. It was supposed to be at the one o'clock position. The gel on the end of the wand might be a little chilly, she explained, though she always tried to warm it up.

I jumped when she pressed the wand to my skin, and set in for a long exploration.

She found it on the first try.

Well, damn.

The machine made little bell sounds as she measured it. Whatever *it* was. She checked the entire breast, including the lymph nodes, while she calmly asked me questions meant to distract me. Was I married? What part of town did I live in? What was New River like? Anything to get me talking and not thinking about the procedure.

After the ultrasound, I adjusted the robe, and she took me down the hall to get the mammogram on the other breast. My technician's name was Joy. Another bit of irony. She was kind and apologetic for the very hard compression that was required to get the views the doctor wanted. Hard compression—that's code for hurts like hell. But I sucked it up and vowed not to scream or cry, and was mostly successful.

When it was over, I found myself back in an empty waiting room with my robe tied tightly around my waist as if it could shield me from further blows to my dignity. I couldn't sit down, I was so anxious. I stood staring out the window but seeing nothing and let my thoughts drift. Just two days before I had attended a memorial service for a friend who had died of breast cancer. My lip quivered as I held back tears.

I thought about all the women I have known who had breast cancer. Some were survivors, and some were—not. I thought about how much I hate the color pink. I thought about how much I didn't want to be a part of the cancer club, thank you very much. I thought about surgery. I thought about radiation and chemo. I thought about losing my hair. Then I thought about holistic treatments I could give myself. I was a healer after all. I thought about the herbs I would take. The meditations I would do. I thought about running away before the nurse came back to get me.

Before I had the chance to follow through, Joy stuck her head in and asked me to follow her to the office where another nurse waited. She told me we were waiting for the doctor.

So far no one had said the "L" word—*lump*—and that was what I grabbed on to. I was scared of the "L" word, and in my mind, I had drawn that as the line in the sand. As long as the doctor didn't use the "L" word, I was okay, there was nothing to worry about. I would go home and resume my life, grateful to the universe, lesson learned.

There was small talk with the two nurses about long marriages and tattoos—I have several of them, including the symbol for the three goddesses on my arm—before the doctor finally came in. She was a well-dressed woman with a compassionate look. She spoke softly as she told me about what looked like calcifications in my left breast. She was patient and kind and didn't use the "L" word. Calcifications, like the white stuff that crusted on our faucets. I could handle that.

Then it happened. She said it.

"We found a lump in your right breast."

The "L" word.

My head swirled. I heard the rest of her comment as if I were underwater.

"It is small…we need to do a biopsy…you'll have results in 24 hours…we'll leave a piece of stainless steel in there to mark the spot in case you have to have surgery."

Surgery.

I felt lightheaded, and I wanted to fly away, but fortunately my training as a naturopath kicked in. I asked good questions and got the information I needed.

The doctor left the room and the nurse remained to go through a checklist of allergies, blood pressure, medications, height, and even weight. I was caught off guard, and I gave her my correct weight. It had gotten late and most patients and staff had already left, but she assured me I would get a call the next day to schedule the biopsy. She handed me a business card, walked me to the door into the hallway, and told me I could get dressed.

I waited for the elevator in a stunned silence. Had that just happened? I looked down at the business card in my hand. Yes it had.

As I walked to the car, my phone buzzed. It was a text from Tom, asking where I was.

I stopped to make the call. I knew my legs weren't sturdy enough to walk and talk at the same time. The first question was, of course, "What happened? How did it go?"

My voice broke. I couldn't tell him like this. "We'll talk when I get home," I said.

I resumed my slow walk to the car, keenly aware that these were the first steps on my new journey. A journey I wanted no part of. A journey I had no choice but to accept.

The drive home was about 25 minutes, and I was able to calm down. Tom had scheduled a trip to New York for a family reunion, and I wanted to make sure he didn't miss that.

Once home I told Tom about the lump and the biopsy.

"What? No," he said. "I'll cancel the trip."

"No, you go. It's no big deal."

"Sounds like a big deal."

"It's a biopsy," I said. "A simple test. I'm a big girl, I can handle it." He wasn't even going for a full week. I assured him that nothing else would be done while he was gone.

"You sure?"

"I'm sure."

And so he went, and I was happy he did.

CHAPTER 2

The saying goes, "When life hands you lemons, make lemonade."

I have a slightly different saying. Mine is, "When life hands you lemons, make a liver flush."

The news that I needed biopsies of suspicious growths in both my breasts brought me very present to the state of my own self-care. In a word, it sucked. And though it sounded to my ears too much like closing the door to the coop after the chickens got away, I decided to do something about it. Experience as an herbalist and naturopath has taught me that a good first step to self-care is a general cleansing of the whole system. And a good first step to cleansing the whole system is to cleanse the organ that does the cleansing—the liver.

I tried not to worry about the biopsies, of course, but they were definitely on my mind, buzzing in the background like the AC unit bolted to our roof. By doing a liver flush, I could tell myself that at least I was doing something proactive for my own care. No matter what the tests would show, giving my liver some TLC couldn't hurt—and it gave me something to do.

I learned the liver flush I use for myself and recommend to my clients over 20 years ago as a budding herbalist from one of my early teachers. It is my tried and true protocol today. And you probably guessed by now it's heavy on the lemons.

The ingredients are lemon juice, orange juice, garlic, gingerroot, and olive oil. You mix them all together, drink it first thing in the morning, and then don't eat or drink anything else for an hour.

The original recipe called for all lemon juice, but I can't stomach that so I add the orange juice to make it taste a little better, at least to me. I have clients who do the straight lemon juice, and they say it tastes fine, but I know my limits. The concoction is actually easier to get down than you might think, but the burp afterwards takes your breath away! Which is part of the point of the liver flush.

A thorough liver flush takes seven days. By the time I had gathered all the ingredients, it was only five days before the biopsies, but I figured that wouldn't be a problem. The office had told me to eat before the appointment. Easy enough. I am an early riser, and I would make sure I did the flush early enough that morning so I could eat before I left home.

On biopsy day, that was what I did. Got up early in the morning—I didn't sleep that much the night before anyway—drank the flush, enjoyed the burp, and puttered around the house until it was time to eat. I had a small breakfast, though I wasn't that hungry. Since Tom hadn't returned from the family reunion, I hopped in the truck with a girlfriend, and drove down I-17 south from New River to the Breast Center.

I found myself back in the room wearing the stylish, yet unsettling robe once again. But at least I wasn't alone this time. I am a strong person, but I wanted someone with me for a couple of reasons. I recommend anyone going through this to do the same.

First, having a friend with me was both comforting and distracting (in a good way)—comforting to have someone to lean on and distracting to have someone to talk to. We chatted about Peaceful Spirit, about what each of us was doing in the afternoon, about the color of the walls. With her there, I didn't feel as if I was facing this alone.

Second, it's good to have someone there to ask the questions you don't ask and remember the things you forget. Appointments like these are highly stressful, and when you are sitting half clothed in a chilly exam room you tend not to be at your best. Your brain shuts down a little. Or a lot. A companion can pick up the slack.

Even with my friend there, I was nervous, but that was to be expected. That was why she was there.

The first biopsy was of the lump in the right breast, and it was guided by ultrasound. The tech locates the lump with the ultrasound wand, and the doctor uses the image on the screen to stick the needle into the lump and take a sample.

The doctor in me was excited they had turned me around in the room so I could see the screen, too. I watched in fascination as the fluid spread throughout the tissue on the screen while at the same time I felt my chest grow numb. Then the needle came into the picture, and pierced the black blob. A lever opened, then closed, grabbing a piece of the mass. I couldn't feel anything, and it was hard to believe the needle was inside me, but it was cool to watch.

Yes, I know I'm weird.

There was a little discomfort, but it was over pretty quickly. The nurse told me to have a seat in the waiting room, and they would get me for the other biopsy, which would be in the room across the hall.

I had been so fascinated watching the procedure I didn't realize I was shaking. My girlfriend hadn't missed it, though. She offered me lavender oil. I gratefully rubbed a few drops on each wrist. Among other applications, lavender has a calming effect.

I really needed the lavender to get through the next biopsy. Not only were my breasts crushed into the machine as before, this time the doctor stuck a needle in the breast for the sample. While I was still clamped in the machine, they x-rayed the sample to make sure they got what they wanted.

They did *not* get what they wanted with the first sample, so they took another one. After twenty minutes in that infernal machine and two passes at the biopsy, I was visibly shaking in pain, and blood was dripping down the machine. The poor nurse kept rubbing my hand and asking if I was all right. I assured her that in fact I was not all right, but that I probably wasn't going to pass out.

Finally, they got a good sample, and it was over. They released me from the compression plates and handed me two little ice packs shaped like daisies. The ice packs lulled me into believing their story that it wouldn't hurt much afterwards—that my breasts might just be a little tender.

Tender, my ass. As the blood flowed back into them, they down right hurt. Bad. They hurt so bad that putting my clothes on was a torture worthy of the Middle Ages.

On the way out, the staff advised me to take Tylenol and said I'd get the results in 24 hours.

After I finally got home I took a nap, watched a marathon of *Diners, Drive-ins and Dives*, and tried not to think.

The next day was Thursday. I was by myself and still very sore. I purposely kept myself busy in the morning and early afternoon. I straightened my office, responded to email, fiddled with my schedule, checked my inventory of herbs and oils.

The doctor had said results usually came in between one and three. From about one on, my cellphone was glued to my hand. I was torn between wanting to know and wanting to pretend this wasn't happening.

I did okay until three, then I found myself looking at the clock every five minutes and then every two minutes, saying "Come on, Doc," as if I could will her into calling in my time frame. One of the great lessons in all this, however, is that no one and nothing really gives a hoot about your time frame. Time has a way of taking charge of you rather than the other way around.

At 3:45 my phone rang. I jumped but answered on the first ring. It was the doctor. *About time*, I said to myself.

After we exchanged greetings, she said, "The lump in your right breast is just a cyst with inflammation. Nothing to worry about there."

Phew, I was thinking. *All that worry for nothing.* I let my guard down. "Thank you doctor—"

"However," she said, talking over my *thank you*. "There is a malignancy in the left breast."

NO! I cried inside my head. *Can't be.*

She kept talking, but my breath was coming in short gasps, and I couldn't make out the meaning of her words. I knew what she was saying was important. I grabbed a pen and pad and scribbled the disjointed words coming through—stage 0…DCIS…remove… MRI…surgeon.

My hand was moving with the name and number of a surgeon. *Surgeon? What? Let's not jump ahead here.*

As much as I had anticipated the call earlier in the day, now I couldn't wait for it to end, and I almost pressed "End Call." But my medical training kicked in, and I asked questions. I asked her to tell me what DCIS stands for.

"Ductal Carcinoma in Situ," she said. "Cancer of the milk ducts."

I didn't like that answer.

"The good news is that it's non-invasive and we caught it early." Good news being relative in these situations. The doctor went on to tell me the surgeon's office didn't close until four, so I still had time to call and make an appointment.

You just diagnosed me with cancer and you want me to make a phone call? Now? All I wanted to do was go back to work and pretend she never called.

I assured her I would call the surgeon—I didn't say when—and ended the call.

I stared at the phone in disbelief.

Did she really just say that I had breast cancer? I looked at the sticky notes all over my desk. Yep, she had said it.

I began to shake. When I realized I wasn't breathing—I was holding my breath as if I had been pulled underwater—I got up from my chair and walked into the treatment room next to my office. I walked circles around the massage table, telling myself to breathe, breathe, breathe. I kept saying it over and over again in my head. Breathe, breathe, breathe. My mantra. It kept me from thinking about what had just happened. What I had just learned. How my life had changed with a single phone call.

I calmed myself with the breath work. I could feel this new information as it passed through all the layers of my being. This was real. This was happening.

I'm not sure how long I paced the floor, but I didn't stop until I felt calm enough to think. Once I found my center, I planned my next steps. There were people to tell, information to gather, and doctors' appointments to schedule.

I didn't want to tell anybody by text or email, for two reasons. One, these seemed like perfunctory ways to tell someone about something so important. And, two, I didn't want to see it in print. If I didn't see it in print, I could pretend it wasn't happening.

It would have to be phone calls.

I called Tom first, of course, but he said he was driving a bunch of people somewhere. "Give me a minute. I'll pull over and call you back."

It only took five minutes, but it seemed like an eternity.

I told him the results, and he was quiet for a moment.

"How do we fix this?" he said. Because that's what he does.

I had nothing really intelligent to offer, since I was blubbering away.

"Do I need to come home?" he said.

"No," I said. "It's only one more day. Enjoy your family. You'll be home soon enough."

"If that's what you want."

"That's what I want," I said, though I wasn't really sure what I wanted. My mind was a little scrambled just then. The best I could say was that that was what I wanted to want.

When my friend arrived at the Center after work, I told her the results, and we hugged and cried for a little.

Now that people knew, it would be much harder to pretend it wasn't happening.

CHAPTER 3

The day after I was diagnosed with breast cancer was difficult. My head ricocheted from thought to thought, and I couldn't concentrate. I hadn't been able to bring myself to call the surgeon. I am a naturopath, and I believe in spiritual and natural healing. Was a surgeon even right for me? What would I do about chemo and radiation? Was the diagnosis correct? Should I get another opinion?

I had all the questions but none of the answers. Fortunately, I only had one client that morning, a massage therapy session. I don't know how, but I managed to get through it without breaking into tears or short-changing the client. At least, I think I did. I hope the client thought so, too. And actually, I do know how I got through it. It's what I do. I take care of other people. So I breathed deeply and focused on the body and soul on the table in front of me, working out the knots of pain and tension. I've always been able to lose myself in working with people, and I came to find that on this journey it was important to continue work, both as a way to channel my energies and, of course, for practical reasons. Bills still have to be paid.

Once I finished with the client, I sat at my desk and did all the follow-up tasks—logged the payment, scheduled the next appointment, looked at my To-Do list. After a bit, I found myself staring blankly at the computer, my head a jumble as it returned to all the questions without answers whirling through my brain. Working with people was one thing, but desk work was another—I needed to get out of the house. I needed to pretend things were normal.

What's more normal than getting a haircut? I called my hair dresser. She had an open slot, and I took it.

The same woman had been doing my hair for almost two years, a young gal whose hair was a different color every time I saw her. We generally talked about anything and everything—my purple hair, her recent wedding, the excitement of owning her first house, our chickens, the Center.

But that day I was quieter than usual, and she asked me how I was doing.

My stomach clenched in pain, and I—couldn't tell her.

The diagnosis was the only thing on my mind, it was central to all my thoughts and feelings, but I couldn't talk about it.

I tried to tell her, but I couldn't say it out loud. I just wasn't ready to make it public.

I lied and said everything was fine, then deflected by asking her questions, which she answered in her usual chatty way.

I let myself off the hook for that small subterfuge. Cancer is such a personal journey that we are the ones who get to decide what to talk about and when. For those out there on the same journey, you don't have to let others set the terms. That's for you and you only.

My trip to town was not just about keeping busy, though. It was also about starting on the next step of my journey. I have supported many other people through health challenges and now it was my turn to take my own advice.

The first thing I did was shop for a notebook. If you follow my blog, you know I recommend keeping a healthcare binder to document everything medical that happens in your life. This is a place to store and record all your medical appointments and their results, all your prescriptions and treatments, whether traditional or alternative, any surgeries or procedures you undergo. It spans a lifetime.

The notebook is different from the binder. It's designed for a single purpose—to record every aspect of this specific diagnosis. You receive so much information, much of it medical and scientific, that there's no way you can keep track of it all in your head. Write it down.

Write it all down, and if you are too overwhelmed to do it yourself, ask a friend or family member to do it for you. Someone you trust to be as detailed as you are. And don't be afraid to sound dumb. If you don't understand something, ask the doctors or nurses to repeat it. Ask them to spell the words you've never heard of. Though some of them don't act like it, medical practitioners work for you. You're the boss. Don't be afraid to act on it.

I wanted a pretty notebook. I wanted something that would make me forget about the diagnosis and why I was buying a notebook in the first place. I went to Staples with its aisle of notebooks and journals, both personal and business. I picked up and opened dozens of possibilities, weighed them in my hands and paged through them. Nothing fit. Not a single one. I stood in Staples staring at the huge selection and cried.

It wasn't supposed to be this way. I had vowed to stay calm and rational about all this.

Fortunately, the store was almost empty and no one saw my tears. I chose a rather plain notebook that would serve my purpose, content with the fact that I could pretty it up myself. I paid the cashier without looking him in the eye and left.

Walking to the car, I pulled the notebook close to my chest and winced in pain, an instant reminder of what I was facing. The biopsy sites were only two days old and still very painful. I never realized how much stuff I pulled into my chest until this happened.

When I got home, I saw that it wasn't such a bad little notebook, and it provided a much needed opportunity to do something practical. First thing, I decorated the cover with stickers of some of my favorite things—butterflies, dragons, hearts, and flowers. Then I had to figure out what I needed to put in it.

This is what I decided to include that afternoon. In the weeks that followed, the pages filled up quickly:

- Doctors: A list of every healthcare professional I encountered and their information—name, address, phone number, and specialty.
- Timeline: A diary of all appointments and interactions to discuss and treat the cancer— the date, the interaction (type of test, phone call, results, and so on), and the healthcare practitioners involved.
- Issues: My honest take on exactly where I was in the treatment plan. A list of things that needed to be addressed for me to achieve optimum health.
- Protocols: All the holistic treatments and practices I did for myself—diet changes, ear candling, energy treatments, herbal recipes, and others listed by date and results.
- Food Journal: Everything I ate and drank.

The notebook also had pockets to hold the loose papers and pamphlets medical offices like to hand out. I planned to take the notebook with me to every doctor appointment and to keep it close at home to write down what I ate and drank.

Putting together the notebook was a diversion, but it was getting to be afternoon, and I still hadn't called the surgeon.

I sucked it up and made the call.

The woman who answered the phone was very matter of fact. "The doctor sees patients on Tuesday and Thursday," she explained to me. "I can get you in next Tuesday."

My mind screamed, "No, that's too soon!" At that point, I had been diagnosed with breast cancer less than 24 hours. I wasn't ready for surgery. I wasn't supposed to be in this club. I didn't want to do this. I wanted to hang up the phone, but instead I calmly replied, "No, Thursday would be better, thank you."

I felt sure she could hear me shaking through the phone.

After a few more phone calls and another request to the insurance company, the pre-surgery MRI was scheduled. I had to make one last call for the day, but as I thought about it, I felt as if I had a lump a of clay in my stomach. She called herself a navigator. Her job was to help me "navigate" breast cancer, as if it were some kind of hike in the mountains. She would explain my diagnosis, tell me next steps, and answer my questions.

She was very nice on the phone, explaining all of this in that warm, friendly, I'm-on-your side way that the best medical practitioners manage so well. But I wasn't buying it. I didn't want a navigator.

Having a navigator meant it was real. It meant I was going to be treated for breast cancer.

CHAPTER 4

The diagnosis of DCIS had been more of a head game than a physical one so far. Physically, I felt no different than I had before the diagnosis beyond the soreness from the biopsies, but emotionally I was on a roller coaster. Though the journey had only just begun, I was already changing my attitude about letting others in.

I pride myself on my independence, on being able to do things on my own, on giving to others without expecting anything in return. But now I had to laugh at the irony of the cancer's location—the left breast. According to energy theory, the left side of the body is the receiving or feminine side; the right side is the giving or masculine side. I'm great at giving, not so much at receiving. A couple of months before this, in fact, the left side of my back had locked up on me. Had that been some kind of warning?

Louise Hay writes about this feminine-masculine balance in many of her books. Her book *Heal Your Body* is the first reference I pick up when dealing with a health issue, and this was no exception. According to Hay (and many others), emotions and mental states are key players in the body's physical health. *Heal Your Body* gives mental causes for many physical illnesses and suggests that new thought patterns can help heal these illnesses.

Hay has this to say about breast problems and cancer: Breast problems are a refusal to nourish the self, that one is putting everyone else first. And cancer represents deep hurt and long-standing resentment. There may be a deep secret or grief eating away at the self.

To help yourself heal, Hay goes on to offer new thought patterns. For breast problems, you should tell yourself, "I am important. I count. I now care for and nourish myself with love and with joy." For cancer, you should lovingly forgive and release the past, to say, "I choose to fill my world with joy. I love and approve of myself."

Yep. I saw myself in these passages. I work hard to deflect things from being about me. Here's a great example. I was telling a friend about my diagnosis, and I said, "It's just DCIS, no big deal."

She looked me straight in the eye and said, "It is a big deal."

I bartered with her. "Okay, it's the littlest big deal you can get."

"Oh, Melanie," was all she could say while she gave me a hug.

Inspired by Louise Hay's teachings, I learned to let people in, slowly but surely. For one thing, with all the medical appointments and procedures, I had to talk to many people and let them tend to me—receptionists, technicians, nurses, doctors, the navigator. For another, the outpouring of love and support that came after my first announcement had been overwhelming. I had no idea so many lives touched mine, and mine theirs. I thank all my friends, and I thank the universe, and if you're going through something like this, I recommend you do, too. Don't lock out friends and family thinking you're doing them a favor. Opening yourself to that kind of love and friendship may well be your first step toward healing.

CHAPTER 5

DCIS stands for ductal carcinoma in situ and means that there are abnormal cells inside the milk duct in the breast. Many physicians and researchers consider it to be the earliest form of breast cancer, while some don't think it should be called cancer at all, since it is not invasive.

Leave it to me to get the cancer no one can agree on.

Most of us are used to hearing about the different stages of a cancer. My DCIS was Stage 0. Pre-cancer, they called it.

When I got the diagnosis, I did the one thing you should probably never do when you are told you have cancer, or any other serious illness, for that matter. I Googled it. The sheer volume of information blew me away. My breath tightened, my heart beat faster, I felt my pulse pounding in my temples. I saw treatment options that ranged from *Take some supplements and you'll be fine* to total mastectomy with radiation and chemotherapy.

I didn't know what to make of it all. No matter what I thought, I could not do this alone.

I booked an appointment with the navigator.

This was my husband Tom's first visit to the Breast Center with me. As we sat waiting for our appointment with the navigator, I tried to distract Tom—and myself. He knew how much I hated pink, and we saw pink everywhere. The scrubs were pink, the shoes were pink, the folders were pink, the décor was pink. I pointed out all the offending pink items I could see.

I wanted to think about anything other than the reason we were there.

When my name was called, Tom stood up with me and caught my elbow as I swayed. I had just stood up too fast, I told myself. My body felt heavy; my feet rooted to the floor. If I followed her through that door, she was going to tell me about cancer. Not just any cancer, my cancer.

Paula had a soothing smile and a steady, positive tone. She seemed to be in her mid-forties, with short hair, and she always wore a pink polo shirt with the medical center's logo on the chest. She showed us into the library. I wasn't prepared for an entire room filled with cancer literature. Everywhere I looked there were books, posters, and anatomy charts. I took comfort in seeing holistic titles in the mix. I pulled my own personal notebook a little closer to my chest as if to shield myself from the other scary books.

We all sat down at a table. It was the first time I noticed the large yellow envelope and notebook Paula had been carrying. The envelope contained copies of my mammograms and results of my biopsies. I would need these for the surgeon.

But the notebook was for me.

It was a three-inch black binder with, you guessed it, pink writing and trim. Surely, she had made a mistake. I couldn't need a binder that big. My cancer was only Stage 0.

She opened it to show me the contents. There was a card from the president of the breast health center, who was a survivor herself. There was a pamphlet about understanding your journey, and then a much larger book called *Be A Survivor.* Paula cautioned me to read only the parts that pertained to my diagnosis. Later I would understand why she said that.

Slowly, the binder gave me some comfort. I could appreciate how far the Western model of medicine has come if practitioners were empowering me with information. She showed me the tab with my imaging results and the pathology reports. Then she showed me the ten other tabs. Not all the sections pertained to me, but all the bases seemed to be covered.

I'll admit I was feeling a little smug. I wouldn't be needing all this stuff. I was a Stage 0, after all.

After she finished with the binder in general, she talked about my specific diagnosis. She explained about DCIS—that it is pre-cancer and Stage 0, which I already knew.

Then she said something I wasn't prepared for.

"Your DCIS is Stage 0, but Grade 3."

Wait. What? No one had mentioned this before.

I knew about cancer staging, but I was not familiar with the grades. Stage runs from 0 to 4 and indicates how far the cancer has spread. Cancer grade, Paula explained patiently, ranges from 1 to 3 and is a function of how fast the cancer cells are dividing.

Mine was the highest grade—Grade 3.

Grade 3 means the cells are growing aggressively.

Growing. Aggressive. Not what I expected to hear given the Stage 0 I had been laying my bets on. It felt like the wind had been knocked out of me.

I struggled to pay attention during the rest of the appointment. I watched my husband's face as he asked very thorough and rational questions to hide his own fear. I was hoping he was getting it all, because I sure wasn't.

Neither of us said anything as we rode the elevator down and walked out of the building. When we got in the car, I cried, secretly, I thought, trying to wipe away the tears without him noticing. He couldn't help but notice. He was looking at me so lovingly.

"We'll get through this," he said taking my hand.

"I know," I replied, though I'm not really sure I believed it just then. It was all so surreal.

He hugged me, and started the car.

We would see the surgeon in two days.

CHAPTER 6

I'm not feeling sick.

I'm not in pain.

I'm no bitchier than normal.

There is only a piece of film and words on a page that say there is breast cancer in my body.

I look the same.

Maybe I don't look the same. Maybe sometimes the mask slips and worry flashes across my eyes.

That's only normal, right?

I'm afraid of the unknown. That's only normal, too, right?

But don't be afraid of me. Please don't be afraid of me. I'm still me. I'm still Melanie. I'm still a healer. I'm still in love with my husband. I still care for my friends and family and clients. I still have a great sense of humor.

Why was I having this crisis of self-doubt?

When I stood looking out the waiting room window at my first appointment, I knew I would be sharing this very personal journey in a very public way. I am a healer and I have a blog, and I knew that I couldn't help but write about this very profound journey. The first writings flowed effortlessly.

And the love poured in.

Emails, texts, social media messages, and cards came in with words of encouragement I hadn't realized I needed. They touched me deeply in a way no words could express.

But then a weird thing happened. The love and concern started to backfire.

Some of my regular clients asked if they should cancel their appointments. One of my clients told me he was not comfortable with me working on him.

"Why?" I asked. He had been a client for years, one of my stalwarts.

"Because you're broken," he replied. "How can you fix me if you're broken?" He admitted that he had wanted to cancel his appointment, but his wife wouldn't let him. *Thank you*, I said in silent prayer.

Broken? Is that what people thought?

After reassuring him that physically I felt no different than I had two weeks before, and that I wasn't broken, maybe just a little bruised, he relaxed and had a great bodywork session.

This kind of awareness has deep implications for a business owner.

I have needs, as a business owner and a human being. And perhaps this is one of the essential differences between Western and alternative medicine. In Western medicine, illness is a weakness. You are "broken," as my client said. Illness is something to be ashamed of, something that needs to be fixed, and if it can't be fixed, you should have the good grace to keep it quiet and hidden. This is an exaggeration, of course, but not much of one. I've heard people say words just like these.

In an alternative, holistic system of healing, however, illness is a stage of life you're going through, another experience, though of course not necessarily a fun experience. There's nothing to hide, nothing to be ashamed of; there's no moral failing to it.

Besides, as a human being, I needed the distraction of work. I needed to feel useful. And as a business owner, I needed the income. I had worked hard to build my business and be of service to the community. The community supported me when it didn't know my personal struggles. Once they knew, I asked them to please continue to support me and the Center.

I've been honest about my challenges with receiving. I'm an independent, do-it-myself kind of woman. I don't like to ask for help. I make up all kinds of reasons why I have to go it alone.

Mostly I'm afraid of being vulnerable. It's almost as if I've backed myself into this corner of constant fear. When did that happen? I have a list of crazy things I did when I was younger without ever being afraid for one single moment.

On a whim, I stopped on the side of the road for a crazy looking trucker who swore he only wanted to look at my map. Then on a bet I married him. Looking back on our 30 plus years together, I would say that act of fearlessness worked out.

Maybe asking for help wouldn't be so bad after all.

CHAPTER 7

The giant yellow envelope was stalking me, I swear. It was so big I couldn't find anywhere to keep it. I tried to move it out of sight—to the top of the filing cabinet, behind the computer monitor, on the book shelf. But every time I sat down to work, or moved around the office, there it was, jumping out at me, a constant reminder of my diagnosis. What was so scary about this giant yellow envelope? It contained copies of the mammogram as well as the biopsy and MRI results—proof that this was really happening. That I really did have breast cancer.

That day I was going to see the surgeon, who needed to examine the contents of that yellow envelope.

My hand shook as I reached for it.

I took a deep breath and tried not to think too far ahead. Then in one swoop I gathered up the envelope and my binder and headed to the truck. Tom was coming with me again.

I had an early morning appointment. The waiting room was empty when we arrived. I worked through the pile of paperwork that I had to fill out when I saw someone for the first time—you'd think in the digital age, it wouldn't be so difficult. When I returned the papers to the receptionist, I tried to hand off the offending yellow envelope, but she told me to hold it for the doctor.

All too quickly we were seated in the doctor's office to wait for the surgeon. She arrived and appeared to be a few years older than I was. She had short hair, wore glasses, and looked extremely smart and competent. When you spoke with her, you felt as if you had her full attention, as if you were the most important person in the world to her just then.

We met in her personal office, not a treatment room. I felt comforted by the things I saw—several binders from breast cancer conferences and framed recognition as a top doctor by *Phoenix Magazine* and *Guide to America's Top Physicians*. All this on top of a friend's glowing recommendation made me breathe a little easier.

I liked her energy as soon as she came into the room. She had a friendly face with compassionate eyes, and was very patient with my questions. I forgot about the envelope in my lap and listened intently to her describing DCIS and my treatment options. She asked if I had a family history of breast cancer. I told her no. That was good, she said. She reminded me that my cancer was at a very early stage and that I didn't need to panic. But she also made sure I understood that Grade 3 meant aggressive growth, and she spelled out why and how this could become more serious.

As she explained the surgical treatment options, including mastectomy and lumpectomy, I felt like someone had punched me in the stomach. This was worse than reading the book.

She told me the standard treatment for my cancer was lumpectomy and radiation. My research had told me as much, but hearing it from the real live doctor who would actually be doing the cutting was surreal. The whole time I was there I felt as if we were talking about somebody else.

We followed her into the treatment room. I remembered the oversized yellow envelope I had been told so many times to bring and held it out to her. She told me that everything was in the reports she had already seen but said, "Let's have a look."

As an anatomy geek, I have always loved looking at radiology films. I've seen my husband's back in an MRI, my mother-in-law's lung and brain scans, countless X-rays of broken bones, MRIs of torn ligaments, and even color pictures of my own ovaries and intestines from appendix surgery. I had kept those pictures on a bulletin board in my room until my husband made me take them down.

I find the human body fascinating and love any chance I get to learn more about it. But that day I didn't feel the same excitement.

It seemed as if there was no end to the contents of that yellow envelope. The doctor just kept pulling out films, holding them up to the lightbox, and pointing out little specks. I saw the clips that were left in my breasts from the biopsies. She reminded me that she would remove the one from my left breast.

I went lightheaded and the color must have drained from my face, because she glanced at me, and promptly turned off the lightbox, saying we had seen enough.

She pulled out a paper top for me to put on as she stepped out of the room. I looked at it with disdain. It was pink, of course.

Feeling vulnerable in the pink paper shirt, I thought about what the doctor had told me as we examined the films. The MRI showed a 5.5 cm area of concern. I asked my husband about the math, and he said it was a little over two inches.

I looked down at my breast. There didn't seem to be enough real estate in there to be taking two inches of anything out. And that two inches didn't include the extra tissue around the DCIS that needs to come out to get clear margins.

I felt my eyes well up. *Will I be disfigured?* I was thinking. *Unattractive? Less of a woman?*

Rationally I didn't think that would be the case, but goaded by anxiety, my mind touched on every bad scenario I could think of. I told myself to just breathe.

The doctor returned and did a quick exam. She told me I was lucky the surgery was going to be on my bigger breast.

Funny, I didn't feel lucky.

She found nothing unusual, and quickly I was dressed again in my own shirt. I couldn't wait to get out of that pink thing.

With my file in her hand she asked, "When do you want to do surgery? I do procedures Monday, Wednesday, and Friday."

Even before the first mammogram, I had had a premonition that I would be having surgery. Because a very close family member had already been scheduled for surgery at the time, I blew off the premonition, thinking I had superimposed myself on the relative's situation. I really liked this doctor, and I already knew that if I truly had to have surgery, she would be the one I chose. But I wasn't ready. I hadn't come to terms with the surgery. And I didn't have all the facts yet.

"Okay," I said. "But I want to meet with the oncologist and radiation oncologist before I make a decision about surgery."

She was surprised. Normally a patient doesn't meet the radiation oncologist until after surgery and then meets the oncologist after radiation. But that was not how I was going to do things. I was a medical practitioner. How could I make an informed decision about the first step in the treatment if I didn't know all the steps and all the players?

The medical assistant was very pleasant as she gave me the referrals. She also seemed compelled to ask if I was ready to schedule surgery. I told her I would get back to her after meeting with the other doctors. I got a surprised look from her as well. I gathered the binder, the big yellow envelope, and the slip of paper that spelled out the names I had to call for the next steps on my journey. Apparently, I was already bucking the system. I smiled at that. If there's one thing I have learned making my way through the American healthcare system, it's to take back as much control as you can. And then some. You have to be your own best advocate.

CHAPTER 8

I fidgeted with the slip of paper in my hand, stared at the two names written there, the names of the oncologist and radiation oncologist. It was hard to believe that little black lines on white paper could create such a physical sensation in my body.

I've been doing energy work for over 15 years. I recognize the power of energy and the interaction with our physical body and have experienced firsthand how emotions can affect health and well-being.

Even so, I was surprised by the energy of cancer. Yes, cancer has its own energy, which I felt very strongly. And it wasn't only the energy of my own cancer. I felt the collective energy of everyone touched by the disease. It was thick and heavy, a strong current with a mixture of fear and urgency that threatened to sweep me away like a flooding river.

And it was easily triggered. I felt its force every time I thought about the cancer, but I usually managed to hold it back. It was when I had to do something about the cancer, however, that this energy threatened to engulf me. That was when I had to fight the hardest.

Once I told the surgeon I would schedule the surgery after I had seen the oncologist and radiation oncologist, I was committed. I had to follow through. I had to schedule those appointments, and that wasn't easy. I laid out the plan in my head. I would see the oncologist in a week and the radiation oncologist the week after. My handwriting was shaky as I wrote the dates and times on the same piece of paper. I was happy with that plan. But I still had to gather up the courage to make the calls. The cancer energy was gaining strength as it swelled toward me, and I was tempted to let it take me away. I didn't have to make those calls today, I thought. I could put them off a week or two, maybe longer. Spontaneous remission was a thing, right? Maybe I'd just wait for that to happen. I felt fine.

Deep down, I knew I couldn't do that. I refused to let the energy sweep me away. I made the calls and set up the appointments as I had planned.

Mine was the first appointment in the oncologist's office that day. I'm an early riser and like to get these things over with. Tom and I had the waiting room to ourselves. I was grateful for the empty room as I got up to walk around and settle my nerves. There was artwork hanging on the walls that had been done by cancer survivors. We talked softly about different pieces while we waited. There were prints of oils and water colors, mostly of nature—birds, trees, oceans—as if all the survivor artists understood that to heal they had to connect with nature. Some of the pictures had religious overtones, and some were just plain freaky. I had no idea what those were about.

A pleasant nurse came to get us. As we followed her, I was surprised at how big the place was. How many exam rooms there were, and how many doctors and nurses were gearing up to start the day. In that moment, I felt the enormity of cancer, how big it could be.

I felt it trying to take away my power.

I took a deep breath and followed the nurse into an exam room. The nurse took my blood pressure and temperature, and asked questions about my paperwork. These activities kept me focused and allowed me to concentrate on things within my control. But then she left, and while we waited for the doctor, the anxiety returned.

The oncologist came into the room with a smile that didn't quite reach his eyes and a firm handshake. He was tall, dark-haired, with a beautiful complexion. He always seemed very well-kept, no matter what time of day I saw him. He paged through my paperwork, confirmed the diagnosis as DCIS, then thumbed through the forms again as if looking for something, shook his head, and asked when I had had the surgery.

"I haven't had surgery," I replied.

"You haven't had surgery?" he asked, perplexed.

I confirmed that I had spoken with the surgeon but had not had surgery.

He put his pen away in his pocket, leaned back in his chair, and said, "Then why are you here?" as if he were scolding me.

I was taken aback. I am an adult, and I was often the one on the other side of the desk. I was not used to being scolded as if I were a child. I had my plan, which I thought was reasonable. Everyone who might be involved in my care would give me their expert opinion, and I would make my decision when I felt I had enough information.

"I want to know what my options are and what you recommend," I blurted out in a voice higher-pitched than normal. I was not feeling as confident as I had when I arrived.

After a look that was not quite disdain, he regained his professional composure and ran it down for me. I was not a candidate for chemotherapy and because the cancer was estrogen receptive, I would be on hormone therapy for five years to reduce my chances of recurrence. He then examined me briefly, ordered some bloodwork, shook my hand and then Tom's, and was off to the next patient. Maybe that person would do it the way he expected.

It was a one-stop shop and the blood draw was done in the same office. As we waited in the hall for the phlebotomist, I could see the place had gotten busy. There was a constant flurry of nurses calling names and patients following them down the hall. The wait for the blood draw was longer than I expected, and in that time I began to worry. Was I doing the right thing? Clearly, this very well-educated specialist in oncology didn't think so, nor had the surgeon, for that matter, though she had been nicer about it.

Inhale.

Exhale.

Let go of the worry.

I *was* doing the right thing, at least for me.

One of the phlebotomists called my name. As I followed her, worry gave way to professional training. I had started my journey in the healing professions as a phlebotomist many moons ago. I watched as she used a butterfly needle to take blood from my arm.

When she finished, she wrapped a purple bandage tightly around my arm and sent me to my husband. He reached past me and pushed open the door marked "Exit" for me to go through. As I brushed past him, I caught the emotion in his eyes, and then I looked out into a waiting room full of people. I was caught off guard by the energy that hit me. I had entered that room with my heart fully open, not guarded at all, but instead of receiving openness and understanding in return, I was hit with the fear and uncertainty of all those anxious people.

What came *through* me at that moment was not *of* me. I was merely the instrument. A huge rush of love went out to all the people in that room. It was bigger than me and made me unsteady on my feet, but I could see its effect almost immediately. No one got up and danced, but most sat a little straighter in their chairs, lost a few lines of tension on their foreheads, and smiled briefly as if to a distant music.

Tom put his hand on the small of my back and guided me out to the hall. I leaned against the wall as we waited for the elevator. *Wow, did that just happen?* I wondered. That wave of love pushing away the cancer energy, if only for a moment. I was softly crying. Neither of us said a word. It was clear from the way Tom held my hand that his heart had also felt that wave of love.

CHAPTER 9

I had learned my lesson with the oncologist, so my defenses were up as I sat waiting in the radiation oncologist's office a week or so later. I had a list of questions and was prepared for the doctor's shock that I hadn't had surgery. I was determined to be stronger this time.

It had been three weeks since I was diagnosed with breast cancer, and some people were shocked that I was, as they put it, "taking my time" deciding on a course of action, as if I wasn't taking this seriously enough. What they called taking my time, I called taking it all in and getting informed. If I had bought into the energy of fear and urgency, I would have already had surgery and radiation by then.

But I didn't feel that same sense of urgency. Ever since I recovered from the initial shock of my diagnosis, I knew I was going to walk this path to surgery. What I didn't quite know was how and when I was going to do that. I refused to fit the mold of the childlike, compliant patient so revered by Western medicine. I would not be rushed through invasive medical procedures and expected to make decisions in a heightened state of stress. That was one of my new rules. Do not make decisions while stressed out.

Before I made such a monumental decision, I wanted to meet all the doctors who would make up the team guiding me through this part of my journey. I hadn't been ready for the pushback from the oncologist, but I was ready for the radiation oncologist.

I like early morning appointments because most of the time the staff are still in a good mood, and that day was no exception. A smiling nurse showed me through the door and guided me to a scale. I made my husband stand so he couldn't see the number as I stepped up. In thirty-three years together, I have never let him know my weight.

Next, we were shown into an exam room, and went through the same routine as all the other visits. They took my vitals and went over the paperwork. One of her routine questions caused me to get emotional: "Is there a history of breast cancer in your family?"

There was no history in the family—until now. My heart hurt as I thought of my sisters and nieces living in the shadow of my diagnosis. I imagined their anxiety as they checked the box that notes a close relative has had breast cancer.

The nurse left. As we waited for the doctor, I held my notebook tightly as if it could give me courage, comforted by all the knowledge I had gathered there.

The defenses I had firmly in place were completely melted by the woman who entered the room. Her energy was so open and her smile lit up her eyes in a way that put me completely at ease. She was tall but sat on a stool that had her looking me straight in the eye.

When I told her I hadn't had surgery yet, she was both surprised and delighted. She commended my good judgment, and we both relaxed as we talked. We talked about DCIS, radiation, HOAs, and chickens. She lived close to the Peaceful Spirit Enrichment Center and was interested in our Labyrinth walks when the weather grew cooler. I liked her.

But we were far apart on one issue—radiation. She recommended a treatment of radiation twice a day for five days after surgery.

My whole body rejected this idea.

There were lots of statistics, she explained. Rational people have done studies. They gathered the data. She made a compelling case without being pushy. I was grateful for that.

I couldn't refute her science, but I trusted my intuition. And my logic. If what I had was pre-cancer that hadn't spread and the surgeon got clear margins when she took it out, then all would be good. What more would be needed? I didn't feel I should get radiation just because I could. I also knew that if I got radiation this time, I couldn't get it again. Shouldn't we just hold on to that big gun in case we needed it later?

As my resistance to the radiation became more obvious, she let me know that we could make a more informed decision after the pathology report came back after surgery. "If it comes back as Stage 1," she explained, "then it would no longer be classified as DCIS and I would highly recommend radiation."

I could feel the color drain from my face. I hadn't realized that was even a possibility. I was a Stage 0, and I had the binder in my lap to prove it. How could she say that? Stage 0 was all I was prepared for. I didn't want to hear this.

She asked if I had thought about when I would have the surgery.

Of course I had. I could hardly think about anything else. I had picked out a date that worked for me, but I hadn't shared it with anyone. If I said it out loud, it would be another step on the way to making this all too real.

I told her the date. I said it out loud.

It was just before she was going on vacation for a couple weeks, so she scheduled me for three days after surgery hoping the pathology would be complete by then. I just wanted to get out of there so I accepted the appointment. She wished me luck and set off down the hall to help another woman navigate her journey. I still liked her.

Later that day I found myself sitting at my desk staring at the phone. I had to call the surgeon's office to set the date. My brain couldn't make sense of it. I didn't feel bad, yet I was going to call someone and ask them to cut into my body and remove a part of me.

But I knew in my heart that this was the right course for me.

I had ridden a roller coaster of emotions. I felt like a failure for not staying healthy. I worried about what others would think. I didn't want to make a big deal about it. I wanted to do it on my own, in the background, to not ask for help. I wanted help, and was blessed by the outpouring of love. I was strong, and I was weak. I was resistant and open. I knew what I wanted, and didn't know anything at all. I'd been scared, and I cried a lot.

And yet there was a place of solidness as well. I had known from the beginning that my journey would include surgery. I knew that I had to be fully present for this experience. I knew this was a pivotal moment in my life.

And perhaps for the first time in my journey that far, I was at peace with that.

CHAPTER 10

I put off calling the surgeon's office for as long as possible. Even though I knew surgery was the right path for me, I was stalling. I didn't want to make the call, and I found all sorts of reasons to put it off. I checked and rechecked my schedule. I talked to my clients and moved things around.

Suddenly, there it was—five full days cleared of interactions and responsibilities.

The date was August 1.

I tried to think up as many positive things about the day as I could. It was the first day of the month, so that meant new beginnings. It was a Monday, so that meant the surgeon and other hospital staff should be well rested. *But what if they hated Mondays?* the negative angel on my shoulder said. What if they were grouchy and hungover?

Breathe and be positive. Breathe and be positive.

It was National Girlfriends Day, and Goddess knows I could not get through this without the help of my girlfriends.

August 1 is also Lammas, one of eight pagan holidays that include the Fall Equinox, Samhain (Halloween), the Winter Solstice, Imbolc, the Spring Equinox, Beltane, and the Summer Solstice. Lammas is the time to celebrate the harvest. The first grain is cut and loaves of bread are baked to celebrate.

I didn't miss the irony of it being a day of harvest.

I called the surgeon's office and told the nurse when I wanted to schedule my surgery. She was surprised that I was making the appointment for three weeks in the future. I assured her that was the best fit for my schedule, and I didn't feel the need to rush. I was calm, cool, and collected—on the phone.

By the time the appointment was set, though, my hands were shaking. I fumbled as I tried to hang up the phone. How come the End button was so damn small? I wanted to blame the phone or anything else for my situation.

But it wasn't the phone's fault.

I had just made an appointment for breast cancer surgery.

Even though I had had the diagnosis for three weeks, it was still hard to wrap my head around it. In that moment, it felt like a big deal. Not just a little big deal, but a stinking whopper of a big deal, the biggest deal I had ever been up against. Holy crap this was CANCER.

As my emotions spiraled out of control, I called on the mantra I was using to get through this: Be Present. Be in the moment.

Being present right then meant being scared. Even though I felt the solidness of my decision, I also felt the fear. One thing I knew for sure was that surgery had not been on my vision board for this year. Slowly, I worked through the jumble of thoughts running through my head, and began to feel calmer. There was nothing to fear at that moment.

But it was coming.

*

Part of the reason I had scheduled my surgery so far out was to be available to help someone else recover from her own surgery. I was grateful for the distraction. I am comfortable being a caregiver and I'm really good at it. Finally, something I could control.

Hers was an invasive surgery with a long recovery time. As I kept track of her medications, made sure she did her breathing exercises, and monitored her food intake, I felt great. I comforted her, spoiled her, treated her, pushed her, and watched her get better every day.

And for a little while I forgot about myself.

The week before my own surgery came way too fast. I listed the things that had to get done before surgery. It was two pages long. I had to finish my blog for posting, move my clients a week out, pay bills, and shop for post-surgery food. I needed chicken breasts, broth, and astragalus (a root) for the ever-powerful chicken soup. I needed bananas, strawberries, apple juice, and greens for green smoothies. I needed chocolate almond milk just because. I wanted to blend some herbal teas. Even though the list looked daunting, I felt pretty confident. I had to work until 8:00 pm the night before surgery, but I got it all done.

Scheduling the surgery so far out was truly a blessing. It gave me time to relax about the decision and lower my state of worry. I practiced being present. I walked the Labyrinth, hung ribbons on the prayer tree, and meditated at the outdoor altar. I found moments of genuine peace in the midst of all this disruption.

I counted down the last week, noting my last Wednesday before surgery, my last Thursday, my last Friday, and so on. I was pretty calm about it. Until Sunday, that is, the day before surgery. That was when I became jumpy in part because I was frantically trying to finish my list, which was more difficult because I couldn't concentrate.

That night I was supposed to take a shower with antibacterial soap. Antibacterial soap is not my favorite for a host of reasons, including the fact that it's bad for the environment, that it could affect the thyroid, and that it helps create antibiotic-resistant bacteria. I took the shower with the antibacterial soap anyway. If you are going to play their game, you might as well follow their rules. Besides, if there was a time I should be bacteria free, it was probably before major surgery.

Tom and I arrived at the surgery center at 8:00 am, and they took me back right away. First, I was to have guidewires put in so the surgeon knew where to go. We took a quick elevator ride to the second floor, and before I knew it I was back in a world of pink—pink robe, pink paint, pink trim around the walls. When I walked into the room, I had a moment of déjà vu, as if I had fallen back to sleep and was having the same bad dream I had just woken up from. Standing there was the same machine, the same nurse, and the same doctor who had done my stereostatic biopsy.

Again I sat in the chair, and again I had my left breast squished between two plates while trying not to pass out from the pain. Both times I'd been there, the nurse was kind. She rubbed my arm and repeatedly asked me if I was doing okay. I wanted to run screaming from the room, but instead I assured her I was fine. I chuckled a little at the thought of passing out and hanging there with my breast stuck in the machine. You have to have a sense of humor.

I got another wheelchair ride back to the surgery center, where I exchanged the robe for an ugly surgical gown and blue hair net. At least five medical personnel asked me what I was having done and examined the stylish white plastic bracelet adorning my wrist. My surgeon came in and asked the same questions, then took out a Sharpie and wrote "Yes" above my left breast. My first response was, Wait a minute. You have to remind yourself what you're operating on? Then I figured, better safe than sorry.

My pre-op nurse was very sweet and apologized for having trouble finding a vein for the IV despite her best efforts. But she was patient and got it on the second try. The anesthesiologist was brief and lacking in bedside manner, but the results were effective. Fluids started running through my IV, and then I was being wheeled down the hall to the operating room, banging the wall as we entered. The room was brightly lit and cold. Two nurses introduced themselves through their sterile gear. I wasn't sure of the proper greeting in these circumstances, so I just said, "Hi."

They helped me hop on the surgical table. Medical geek that I am, I was excited to look around the room, though the two giant lights above my chest partially blocked my view. I wanted to ask questions about all the fascinating equipment I saw, but I thought better of it. I didn't want them distracted from the work at hand. The anesthesiologist covered my mouth and nose with a mask, my wrist started to burn, and that was the last I remembered until…

…I woke up shaking violently. The post-op nurse came over and told me it was from the anesthesia and gave me something in the IV that calmed it down. I was drowsy and a little nauseated, but Tom and my girlfriend were there telling me they loved me and helping me wake up. It wasn't long before I was dressed and in the car.

I don't remember the drive home. I know that later in the day, I ate some soup, took my pain medication on schedule, and drifted in and out of sleep. That was the routine for two days.

On the third day, I was more alert and hungry, and I was able to sit up in a chair to watch TV when my cellphone rang. It was my surgeon.

"Well, I have good news and not so good news," she said.

I fumbled with my phone to put it on speaker so Tom could hear as well. I sat up straight and listened intently.

"The good news is that there is no sign of the cancer growing outside the duct. So it was contained."

That does sound like good news, I said to myself.

"The not so good news is that we didn't get it all. The margins weren't clear, and we need to take out more tissue."

Yep. That wasn't such good news all right. I would need a second surgery.

I couldn't say anything. Thank goodness Tom was there to take over the conversation and ask questions. Her voice sounded far away as she explained the additional amount of tissue she would need to take out, that she would use the same incision, and that it was better to do this sooner rather than later. I should call the office to schedule the next surgery. Her tone was empathetic, and she was patient with our disbelief.

But that hadn't changed what she said.

After we hung up, I laid the phone on the table and felt a wave of sadness wash over me.

Another surgery. This was not what I had expected.

CHAPTER 11

I was rocked by the news that I needed another surgery. Even though the doctor had warned me that 20% to 30% of women require a second lumpectomy, and a friend had told me she had had two lumpectomies herself, for some irrational reason I had thought I would be one and done.

I was to have two lumpectomies in eight days.

I wasn't dragging it out this time. From a physical standpoint, I thought it was better to schedule the second surgery quickly. I wanted my body to have the best possible healing, so I considered things like scar tissue, anesthesia, stress, and the fact that I wanted to get it over with.

All of my work appointments the week after my first surgery were tentative, so I moved them to the next week and tried not to worry about how I was going to pay the bills.

The second surgery was scheduled for Monday. I would be having surgery two Mondays in a row.

I was really starting to dislike Mondays.

I woke up from the first surgery wearing what they call a binder. Think a white tube top with a wide Velcro strip down the front to hold it together. When I first saw it, I flashed back to my teenage years when tube tops were all the rage and I was a bit thinner and actually looked good in one.

At the time I found out I needed a second surgery, I still hadn't seen anything but the bandage over the surgery site. Gauze covered the incision, and a clear waterproof bandage covered a large portion of the breast. I had tugged opened the Velcro to look at the breast when I got home, but it hurt without the binder, so I tightened it back up and left it alone.

I only took the binder off to shower. After a couple of showers, the waterproof bandage peeled back around the edges. Even though my breast was still swollen and tender, I gently picked at the edges of the clear bandage to see if I could get it off. The more I pulled at the bandage, the more my hands shook.

I was scared of what I would see under that bandage.

The clear cover peeled away more easily than I expected, and the gauze suddenly fell away from the incision. I gasped and stared at what I saw in the mirror.

It looked like an art project gone very badly wrong.

The incision followed the edge of the areola on the side closest to the arm and was crossed by nine Steri-Strips radiating inward, terminating at the nipple like half a daisy. There was a blue line around the areola where the surgeon had marked her cut, a faint outline of the "Yes" she had written before surgery, two holes from the guidewires, and bruises on both sides of the breast colored blue and green and yellow.

And it hurt.

After a few minutes I breathed again and reminded myself to be present. I can handle this, I told myself. I can handle this. I summoned all the professional objectivity I could muster, and I looked at my breast again in the mirror, this time able to appreciate the complexity and precision of what my surgeon had done. Over the next few days I kept Tom and my girlfriends up to date on the breast art project. It was like being a teenager again. All you had to do was ask, and I'd pull up my shirt and show you my breast.

Each day I got a little healthier, and each day I got closer to another surgery.

This surgery was scheduled for 1:45 in the afternoon. That wasn't optimal. I couldn't have anything to eat or drink after 3:45 am. I set my alarm for 3:30, got up, and drank a crazy amount of water. I didn't want to be dehydrated when the nurse went looking for a vein the next day. I was scheduled to coach a client on the phone that morning. I was grateful for that appointment. We worked well together on that call, and the hour flew by too quickly.

Again, I had to focus on me.

My family was thoughtful and didn't eat in front of me. I tried to keep busy puttering around the house, but I looked at the clock way too many times. The time plodded on, dragging like—well, like I was waiting for surgery.

Tom and I were quiet on the car ride to the surgical center. I think we both had the feeling that, now that we knew what to expect, we just wanted to get it over with. Walking into the building gave me an uncomfortable feeling of déjà vu. Or was it déjà déjà vu? I couldn't tell, I had been there so many times now.

The woman at the registration desk said I looked familiar. I told her she had checked me in last Monday for the same surgery. She said something intended to comfort me and wrapped another stylish white plastic bracelet around my arm.

I sat nervously waiting for the nurse to call my name. I shuddered, and Tom reached over to hold my hand. My stomach was doing flip-flops as the fear and doubt rose within me. I drew in a deep breath. Breathe, I said to myself. Be present.

A nurse came through the door and called my name. She checked my bracelet to make sure it was me and told my family she would come and get them once she got me prepped. They hugged me as tightly and told me everything was going to be okay. I gathered my courage and followed the nurse through the door.

Again I hit the jackpot when it came to nurses. She was kind and shared my feelings of injustice at having to come back for a second surgery. My vitals were good and nothing had changed since last week except for, you know, that incision on my breast.

I was close enough to the computer to see the information on the screen. I was watching her type in my blood pressure when I noticed a little red check toward the bottom of the page. It was the only red on the page, so my eyes went right to it. The red check mark was next to the word *cancer*. My eyes welled up with tears. You'd think by then I'd remember I had cancer and wouldn't react so strongly to a simple word. But time and again through this journey the word *cancer* struck me like a blow.

The idle conversation between the nurse and me turned to my work as an herbalist. The more I told her about my training and the Peaceful Spirit Enrichment Center, the livelier our conversation became. She was interested in herbs and told me she had ordered some Arnica oil for the pain from a recent tooth extraction. I recommended other herbs she could use with the Arnica oil. She pulled out a pen and wrote them down.

Another nurse came by and asked if this nurse needed any help. She said no but excitedly told the second nurse about my herbal background. Her eyes widened and she asked if I taught classes. "Why, yes, as a matter of fact I do," I said. She got called away but promised to come back to learn more about the classes.

Talking about herbs kept my mind off the needle she had stuck in my hand for the IV and the hairnet and hospital socks that meant another trip to the operating room. The second nurse returned and told us how she had met Rosemary Gladstar (a world-renowned herbalist) at an event in Maine. By the time my family came back to join me in pre-op, the room was filled with women talking about plants. It's not often you get to feel strong and knowledgeable as a patient in a hospital, and I relished the moment.

The doctor was running late, and she was surprised the room was so full. A little smile touched her face when she felt the light and love there. But business was business, and her business was cutting me open. Again she whipped out the Sharpie and wrote "Yes" on my chest above the left breast. I teased her about how long it takes to get that off.

The doctor said this would be a short procedure, and because it was so late in the day, we shouldn't expect the pathology report until Thursday. She would call me when she received it. Both nurses came by to see me before they took me to the OR, one to say good-bye because her shift was over and the other to tell me she would be waiting for me in recovery. Oh, right. I was headed for another operation. I had almost forgotten why I was there. Almost.

I woke up this time without the violent shakes. True to her word, my nurse friend was waiting for me and helped me make a smooth transition to alertness. A little apple juice, and some help getting dressed got me out the door in no time.

At home, binded and bandaged once again, I knew how to stack the pillows and gently place ice on my breast so I could start down the road to recovery. I ate something light and went to bed early. It had been quite a day. I had to get up during the night to take some pain medication, but the leftover anesthesia helped me fall back to sleep.

I remembered how Tuesday was going to go. Regular doses of pain meds and lots of naps. I kept the ice close by and told myself that I was already healing faster than last time.

I was startled awake by the phone just before 4:00 pm and puzzled when the caller ID showed the name of my surgeon. Tom handed me the phone, and I answered it.

As soon as she started talking, I knew it was too much for me. The surgeon wasn't supposed to call until Thursday. My medicated brain tried desperately to understand what she was saying. I put the phone on speaker so we could all listen.

She told us the pathologist had called her already, but the news was not good. Not only did we not have clear margins, there was evidence of a microinvasion—cancer cells found outside the duct.

The cancer was spreading.

I would need a third surgery, and this time she would have to take a lymph node out. She said that I should consider a mastectomy.

No, not a mastectomy! It felt as if all the air had been sucked out of the room. I struggled to breathe. I shook so hard I dropped the phone, which Tom picked up and held. I listened silently as she told us the details of the test results. Her words were hard to hear over the voice screaming in my head, "This isn't fair! This isn't fair! This isn't fair! I did everything right. This isn't fair!"

I tried to understand everything she said, but all I really wanted to do was hang up, curl into a ball, and pretend she hadn't called.

Finally, she told me to keep my appointment with her the following week and said goodbye.

I slumped to my knees and cried uncontrollably—a deep heart-wrenching cry that made my whole body shake. I crossed my arms over my chest as wave after wave of emotion crashed over me.

When my awareness returned to the room, I could feel arms wrapped tightly around me, holding me while I cried on the floor. I looked up and saw two faces filled with tears and the most compassion and love that can flow between beings.

No matter what I thought sometimes, I was not in this alone.

CHAPTER 12

From the moment I was diagnosed with breast cancer, I had a deep knowing that I was supposed to walk this path. It was significant. How could it not be? There was a lesson in this for me, a very profound lesson.

I knew I was nowhere near the end of the journey, but I was already living part of that lesson.

I was not unlovable. I was feeling love beyond measure.

Most of my life I have struggled with feeling unlovable, maybe because of my childhood. I had a pretty rough childhood. I learned early on that if I was going to survive I would have to make my own way, would have to be strong and brave and independent. Now anyone who has had a tough childhood understands that on the other side of that coin are deep feelings of self-doubt, unworthiness, and fear of abandonment. You crave connection, but you don't want to be weak, you don't want to be hurt, so you close down, you shut out all but the most important people—and sometimes even them. I have learned to let Tom in, to let in my best friends. I have learned to balance the feelings of hopelessness with love and gratitude, but I have to stay vigilant.

But here was my lesson. Cancer was cracking me wide open.

In the midst of so much uncertainty, I had never felt so solid, so loved.

I was learning to receive with grace.

Grace came in the form of phone calls, emails, text messages, social media posts, blog comments, donations, and greeting cards. I was blown away by the outpouring of support.

Though all of these messages touched me, there was something particularly magickal in the greeting cards. The cards have been coming in since I was first diagnosed. They came in every size and shape. Some were handmade, and others store bought. They were adorned with flowers, dragonflies, fairies, dragons, the sun, the moon, and the stars. But as with people, it was what was on the inside that touched my heart. Each card had a handwritten message of love and support that made my eyes well up with tears. They filled the empty places in my heart, those hollowed out by all the fears of those of us with tough childhoods, with the love I'd never thought I'd deserve.

I used them to get through the hard stuff. Whenever I felt overwhelmed or beaten down, I picked up that stack of cards and paged through them. They inspired me to keep going. After all, I couldn't let these friends and loved ones down. I had to repay their faith and love. I had to fight, and I had to win the fight. For me and for all those pouring forth their love.

I went to the follow-up appointment as the surgeon instructed, accompanied by Tom and my girlfriend. She told me again that the test results from my second surgery were not so good and that I had more hard decisions to make. I was really getting tired of being a grown up. At least I got to wear my own clothes.

I had already read the pathology reports from both surgeries, so my adult brain understood what she was telling me, but the little girl inside me was stomping her foot and pouting. Why me? I'd done what had been asked of me. Why weren't things turning out the way I wanted them to?

As we talked, pains shot through my left breast, as they did whenever I had a serious conversation about the breast. They were quick little pains that varied in intensity from barely noticeable to so sharp they made me gasp. I felt the same pains when I got overly tired. This reinforced my understanding of how thoughts affect our physical bodies.

The surgeon patiently answered all our questions. I still liked her, but I sure didn't like the things she was telling me. She estimated she had taken out tissue about the size of a silver dollar that was half an inch thick. I complimented her on her skill because I couldn't tell any difference in the size of my breast. She burst my bubble—almost literally—when she told me the area was filled with fluid that would drain away as I healed, and that areas of the breast would eventually cave in.

After all the questions and answers, all the information and data, it was up to me. Did I want a third lumpectomy with lymph node removal or a mastectomy?

I didn't want either, really. But that wasn't one of the choices.

Back in the office, the doctor's surgical assistant handed me business cards for plastic surgeons who could do the reconstructive surgery after a mastectomy—just in case. She suggested I call them to see which ones were covered by my insurance. Without looking at the cards, I put them in my binder and headed for the door.

We were all silent as we walked to the car and got back on the road home. It was only 10:00 am, but we had already suffered a major disappointment.

Once we were underway, I took a deep breath and opened the binder to check out the business cards. One moment I was comparing the information on their cards, all rational and logical, completely in control, then suddenly I burst into tears, startling Tom as he drove.

"Are you okay?" he asked softly.

"I can't believe I am even thinking about having my breast cut off. How did I get here?"

I sobbed uncontrollably. My girlfriend touched my shoulder lovingly and handed me a tissue as tears plopped in my lap.

This couldn't be happening.

When we got home, I called the plastic surgeons while I still had momentum and found that none of them took my insurance.

The insurance company's website was no help either, so I decided to call them directly and ask for names of plastic surgeons who took the insurance.

A young man took my call and my voice shook as I told him I was looking for surgeons who do breast reconstruction after a mastectomy. He politely asked to hold while he checked. After a brief silence, he returned to ask if I had pen and paper.

My pen was poised to write as he gave me the first name: *Affiliated Dermatology.*

What?

"No," I tried to explain. "I'm looking for a plastic surgeon."

"They list plastic surgery as one of their specialties," he replied.

I tried politely three more times to help him see how a dermatologist was not what I needed whether or not plastic surgery was one of their specialties. Finally my frustration got the better of me and I blurted out, "Listen, there is a huge difference between taking off a mole and reconstructing a breast!"

He was quiet for a moment, then said quietly, "Ah, yes."

I wasn't sure if he got it or he just didn't want me to lose it again. He gave me the names of two plastic surgery centers and one private practice. I took these down, showing only my best behavior, and thanked him for his help.

I hate losing control like that, and I had been shaking so bad, the notes on the paper were hard to read. I rewrote what I remembered to make it legible, but had to go online to make sure I got it right. Two of the three mentioned reconstruction; one listed only augmentation.

I felt the sadness getting heavier with each click of the mouse.

I read descriptions of the surgeries, freaked out at the recovery times, and looked at the before and after pictures. I didn't like any of the after pictures.

My brain was reeling. Fortunately, I had a client that afternoon. I set aside my thinking mind and let my higher Self take over. We had a great session, and I was able to politely deflect her questions when she asked how I was doing.

I wasn't sure I could hold it together if I had to talk about my own stuff.

Afterwards, I felt more grounded and was able to tap into my training to sort things out. I have always believed that when it comes to healing we should do the least invasive things first. I love my breast and wasn't ready to give it up. So even though it would be for the third time, a lumpectomy felt less invasive to me.

I reached over to the corner of the desk and picked up the stack of greeting cards. I flipped through the colorful pile, opening some to read the messages and gently touching others just to admire their beauty. I breathed deeply, and made my decision.

I made a few phone calls back and forth with the surgical center, and scheduled my third lumpectomy. On yes, another Monday. Did I say how much I hate Mondays?

CHAPTER 13

There is a Latin phrase, *"omne trium perfectum,"* which means everything that comes in threes is perfect. Or as we say in America, "Third time's a charm." That was my mantra on the Monday morning when I went in for my third lumpectomy.

This was my final chance, and it had to be perfect.

I felt like a celebrity when I arrived at the surgery center. Everybody recognized me or my family. The elderly volunteer who worked the information desk greeted Tom like they had known each other for years. The woman working the registration desk expressed her condolences for my return.

I took an all too familiar seat in the lobby and waited for my name to be called. Emotionally I was having a much harder time with this surgery, maybe because I knew exactly what to expect. That's not always a good thing. Who really wants to know how much pain you're going to feel every step of the way?

It had also been fourteen days since my last surgery, the last Steri-Strip had fallen off, and I finally had a day where I didn't really need a nap. I was just beginning to feel like myself, and here I was at the surgery center again. I was emotionally exhausted, tired of having to make such big life—and, let's face it, death—decisions, and scared of the scars that might be left behind, both physical and emotional.

After that day's surgery, I would end up having had three surgeries in 22 days. Not something I would recommend, but you couldn't fault me for procrastinating any more. I was committed.

The lobby was full that day, and every one of us shared the energy of uncertainty and hope. We all passed the time in our own ways. Some talked quietly with their companions, some read books or magazines, others kept still and quiet with their thoughts. I said a silent prayer that this would be my last time there.

When my name was called I took a deep breath before rising, then I stood up tall and gathered my energy. A round of hugs from the family sent me out of the room feeling loved and protected even more.

As I approached the nursing assistant who had called my name, I saw a quizzical look on her face. I could tell she thought I looked familiar but couldn't place me. "Third surgery this month," I told her. She looked shocked and relieved that she had a good memory and wasn't going crazy. No, that was me. For her, I was one of hundreds of patients who passed through the office every day, every week, every month. For me, this was my one and only breast surgery center. I knew every inch of the office and exam rooms, and these people who had been strangers just a month ago were now almost family.

As if to prove my point, just a few steps into pre-op I heard an excited voice shout my name. My nurse friend with an interest in herbs. "I recognized your name on the schedule this morning and was excited I was going to see you," she said as she gave me a big hug. "But sad you have to come back."

"Me too," I said, returning her hug.

"I've got to finish up with another patient, then I'll be back to take care of you." She headed down the hall.

If I had to be there, at least I was among friends.

The nursing assistant took my vitals. I was surprised to see my blood pressure was higher than it had ever been before. She recorded the information, gave me a gown and slippers, and pulled the privacy curtain as she left. As I stood there alone, I had a moment of panic. Was I doing the right thing with this third lumpectomy?

I took a deep breath, and found my courage again. I had considered the risks and options, and this is what I came up with. Besides, it was kind of late to do anything else about it now.

I changed my clothes and hopped into the bed and laughed. A good sense of humor is critical in these situations. I was thinking that no matter how many times I wore this outfit— hospital gown and non-skid slippers—I couldn't get used to it. It just wasn't the fashion statement I wanted to make to the world, and I never quite felt warm enough.

I snuggled under blankets that had come straight from the warmer and tried to stop shivering. I wasn't sure if it was nerves or the cold room.

The pre-op was as busy as the lobby. I waited a while before my nurse friend came in wearing a big grin. My face lit up in response. We talked briefly about the injustice of a third surgery, and she asked all the required questions as efficiently as possible. I asked how she was healing from her tooth extraction. She told me what herbs she had used and how well they had worked and thanked me for my advice. She also let me know that the other nurse who shared our passion for herbs was on duty. She would come by to see me as soon as she was free.

We got down to business. It was time for the IV. I told her that the back of my hand was still not feeling right from the last IV and there was a flat spot in the vein where the needle had been inserted. She tried to find another insertion point, but my veins were not cooperating. We just couldn't find the right spot. Finally, we agreed to try the back of my hand again but to stay away from the previous insertion.

We both knew when the vein blew. She had hit it fine, but the spurting blood told us it had been too weak. "You're going to have a bruise," she said, pressing the wound with a fold of gauze to stop the bleeding.

"It'll match my boob," I laughed.

My second nurse friend came in and we exchanged excited greetings. Her timing was perfect, since she is the nurse they call for the hard sticks. The three of us talked about herbs and other fun things while my hand got bandaged up and she looked for another vein. The choices weren't good and she tried one on the inside of my forearm.

It hurt when she stuck me, and they both were concentrating on it intently when it blew, too.

Damn. That's gonna leave a mark, I remember thinking.

I already had two bandages and still didn't have an IV in place. The next stick was successful, but they both felt bad about the bruising. I assured them I understood—my veins just didn't want to be there that day. I couldn't say I blamed them. And I didn't miss the irony of getting stuck three times for my third surgery.

When the doctor arrived, the room was filled again with family and nurses. She laughed when I asked if there was any chance she was having a buy 2, get 1 free sale.

We went over the procedure. It was going to be more invasive this time, with two incisions, the same cut around the areola, and an additional cut into the armpit to get the lymph node. I would be injected with dye to lead the surgeon to the Sentinel Lymph Node, as it was called, that she would take out to be biopsied. When I got home, I would pee blue.

That was new.

When the doctor had answered all my questions, she pulled out her Sharpie and wrote the all too familiar "Yes" on my left breast. You'd think she would have figured it out by now.

The nurse came to get me for the operating room, and I said my goodbyes. She unlocked the bed and asked if I was ready. No, I told her. I didn't have my blue hat. She dug around under the pillow and handed it to me. I knew the routine all too well.

I forced myself to breathe deeply as she wheeled me down the hall. I was more scared this time. It had to be the last time. It just had to be.

I woke up with some pain that was quickly managed as I struggled to focus. I had asked the anesthesiologist before the surgery to use whatever they gave me for the second surgery because I hadn't felt nauseated when I woke up. Thankfully, he had listened. I did not feel nauseated.

Since I felt pretty well—relatively speaking, of course— Tom helped me dress, and I was out of there as soon as possible. I gave my nurse friend in recovery a hug and said good-bye.

At home, I took up my healing routine, with the ice pack, pain medicine, and sleeping nest. I had gotten this part of it down pretty well. I slept through the afternoon, night, and most of the next day in that post-op half-sleep that some of you are familiar with, I'm sure; when you don't know if you're dreaming or awake, and you think you're having phantom conversations.

I emerged from this state about mid-afternoon the next day and was awake, more or less, at 4:15 pm when the phone rang. The caller ID indicated it was the surgeon's office. The last time she had called this quickly, it had been bad news. I was in a panic as Tom answered the phone. He put it on speaker.

The surgeon identified herself and said, "The third time's a charm. We got clear margins and the lymph node was negative."

I was speechless. There were no words that could express the emotion I felt in that moment. So I cried.

I found my voice and thanked her. She said she would see me next week at my follow-up.

Tom and I sat for a moment just staring at the phone, tears of joy streaming down our faces.

No more surgery.

CHAPTER 14

Apparently, when the doctor told me my surgery results were good, my brain understood that I was done, finished, everything was back to normal, and I could get on with my life, pick up where I left off.

That, however, was not the case. My brain wanted to party, but my body was saying not so fast. I had had three surgeries in 22 days. In fact, the last surgery had been the most painful because of the additional incision in the armpit to remove the lymph node.

I settled for enjoying my happy brain and nurturing my injured body.

We had a system.

I was back in the recliner nest. I was a pro by then at how to stack the pillows just right so the icepack could contact the injured parts without hurting. Tom placed a pitcher of water where I could reach it, and every time I took a pill one of us recorded it on the refrigerator.

But this time was different. My whole shoulder hurt, top and bottom. Do you know how often you use the muscles in your arm pit? Often, I am here to tell you. Every time I moved it even a little, it tugged at the incision and hurt. Every time I tried to stretch my arm over my head, it brought tears to my eyes.

I felt broken. When I looked at myself in the mirror, I saw that familiar half-daisy pattern of Steri-Strips around the breast, but now an additional row of strips covered the two-inch incision under my arm. I had to take several deep breaths to keep me from the panic that rose whenever I saw my poor mauled breast. I felt as if I moved my arm the wrong way, I'd damage something permanently.

But I am nothing if not stubborn, as you may have come to realize by now. I had come too far to let this get me down. I rededicated myself to healing and mobility. I stretched my arm over my head and did range-of-motion exercises as often as I could stand it. Even more. It hurt, I won't lie, and I whined a lot and made a lot of other noises I'm not proud of—grunts and groans, and screeches. But I did it. I forced myself. I had swum more than halfway across the river to healing and I refused to give in then. That is not how I live my life.

You would think after three surgeries the hard decisions would be over, but there was still another Monday to dread. My appointment with the radiation oncologist was the Monday following surgery.

When I first learned of my diagnosis, I bucked the medical system by meeting with radiation oncologist and oncologist before starting *any* treatment. That's not how it's usually done. Normally a patient doesn't meet with the radiation oncologist until after surgery.

I was grateful I had taken the time to meet with her before I started treatment because I was not at my best when I saw her after the surgeries. And I was not prepared for the energy I found there.

My original diagnosis was DCIS Stage 0, Grade 3. When I first met the radiation oncologist I told her I did not believe radiation was a good choice for me. I reasoned that if everything was taken out with surgery I would not want to further damage my body with radiation.

There I was three surgeries later with a micro-invasion that upgraded me to Stage 1, and even the surgeon was advocating radiation. It is, after all, the conventional treatment.

But I am by no means conventional.

With every surgery, I had felt a solidness when I made the decision. I had been scared, but grounded. Once I decided the course of action, it had felt right.

The very thought of radiation caused my breathing to grow shallow, my heart to beat faster, and my stomach to hurt. There was no solidness there. No feeling that this was the right thing.

Still, I struggled with the decision. Part of my logical side thought that maybe everyone else was right. That if I did radiation now, I could zap this cancer for good. Besides, things were different; the DCIS had been more widespread than originally thought, and there was a micro-invasion. Maybe radiation *was* the way to go.

On the other hand, the surgeon had said we got the clear margins and the lymph node was negative for cancer cells. Why subject myself to strong doses of radiation if I didn't have to? Maybe my gut was right, and radiation wasn't necessary.

I did more research and looked at the statistics. I talked to women who hadn't gone through radiation. I talked to women who had gone through radiation. Still, every time I thought about radiation, my stomach hurt.

I meditated at the outdoor altar, walked the Labyrinth asking for guidance, and tied more ribbons to the prayer tree. No matter how I looked at it or meditated on it, radiation just didn't seem like the right path. I never got that this-is-right feeling.

By Sunday, I made a decision and felt strong about it. I would NOT have radiation.

I knew this was the right decision for me, but I'd have to be strong in the face of the "authorities." I practiced my resolve as Tom drove me to the doctor's office Monday morning.

My radiation doctor's office is literally across the hall from the surgery center. As we went in, I thought for a moment about stopping over to see my nurse friends, but then I figured I'd get distracted and lose my edge.

When I first met this radiation oncologist we had talked about our chickens and how she loved fresh eggs. That morning we sat in the waiting room with a six pack of fresh eggs for her. I smiled as I thought about a time when country doctors would take eggs as payment for services. Those days are long gone.

My name was called, and Tom and I followed the nurse back to an exam room. I was excited when the scale revealed I had shed ten pounds. This is not the way I recommend losing weight, but it was definitely a bonus.

After the nurse left we waited for the doctor to arrive. Tom and I chatted nervously about nothing. There is an unmistakable, heavy, anxious energy about cancer, and it was palpable in this doctor's office.

The doctor walked in wearing a long skirt and a smile. She thanked us for the eggs and shared a short story about her family raising chickens when she was a kid. I liked her as a person and felt confident in her skill.

She looked me straight in the eye and said, "Wow! Three surgeries. Are you ready to start radiation?"

My stomach lurched, hurting immediately. Inside my head I screamed, "NOOOO." But with my outside voice I just quietly said, "I don't want to do radiation."

Over the next few minutes, the doctor did her job exceptionally well. She told me about the risk factors and other scary statistics if I declined radiation, all to convince me to follow the conventional wisdom, of course. She used terms like "survival rate" and "chance of recurrence" that had an immediate impact on my energy.

I got scared.

What if she was right? What do I know? I'm a naturopath. She's a radiation oncologist. I've never done this before. She's done it hundreds of times, probably thousands.

She recommended whole breast radiation, once a day for four weeks.

I asked about the brachytherapy option, where they insert a catheter inside the breast and radiate from the inside. Wait. I didn't want that either. Why was I even asking?

I shook with fear and doubt.

She wanted to see the size of the cavity in my breast from all the surgeries. A technician came in and whisked me off for a quick CT scan. All I needed to do was slip my arm out of the paper shirt and lay on the table with my arm over my head.

Easier said than done.

It still hurt a lot to raise my arm over my head. Keeping it there for the duration of the scan was a real test of my pain tolerance. And

I wasn't winning. There were tears in my eyes as she pulled me out of the machine.

I needed help to lower my arm and I dried my eyes as she led me back to exam room to wait for the doctor. I was visibly shaken when I arrived, and Tom asked if I was okay.

"Should I do this?" I asked him desperately. My armor was cracking under the fear of the unknown.

Fear flashed in his eyes before he said all the right things to calm me down.

"I love you."

"You're the strongest woman I know."

"You know best what's right for you."

"Go with your gut."

"Did I say I love you?"

The doctor returned with a black and white picture in her hand. "Are you sloshing?"

"What?" I replied.

"You have an air pocket in the space where the fluid is and some women report a sloshing sensation when that happens."

I assured her that I was not sloshing.

She held out the picture and explained what we were looking at: ribs, heart, lungs, right arm, breast tissue, and a gray half circle with a black triangle above it on my left breast. This is the cavity created by the surgeries—the gray is fluid, the black the air pocket. The cavity is the size of a 2" x 2" cube, she explained. And I should expect to lose one to two cup sizes in that breast.

What? I couldn't afford to lose that much. I was up to only three to start with.

I felt the familiar pains that pierced my breast when I talked about it. My heart hurt, and I wanted desperately to wake up from this horrible dream.

She went on to explain how precise radiation was these days and that modern technology allowed them to inflict less damage on the surrounding body than in the past. On the other hand, one side effect would be that the ribs on that side would grow more brittle. Too much coughing or too strong a bear hug could crack one of those ribs.

She continued her case for whole breast radiation. When she was done, I asked if all that meant brachytherapy was not an option.

No, it was still an option, and on the plus side, it could cause scar tissue to help fill in the cavity so I wouldn't have as much disfigurement.

I wanted to run out of the room.

I tried desperately to find that rock solid resolve I had against radiation when I had left the house this morning. I was no longer sure of myself. Any power I had was slipping away.

I was so overwhelmed, I disengaged, shut down. The doctor asked when I was to see the surgeon for a follow-up. The next day, I told her. She advised me to talk with the surgeon about it, and then call the office to schedule the radiation.

I asked her for the picture.

As I rose to leave, I was unsteady on my feet. Tom took my hand to steady me, and we walked quietly to the car.

I sat looking at that black and white picture in my hand and burst into tears. I was so confused, but I had felt so confident and solid when I left the house this morning.

Now what should I do?

CHAPTER 15

I was disappointed in myself. I had not expected to lose my nerve when I saw the radiation doctor. I really wanted to be that strong, empowered woman who knows her own destiny.

Whatever.

I was doing the best I could.

The further I got away from that doctor's office, the stronger I became. I regained control of my energy and began to breathe again.

I would NOT do radiation.

I still knew in my heart that it was the right decision for me. And as much as I didn't want to make all these hard decisions, I knew that no one else could make them for me.

I was not scared of dying, but I was scared of making poor choices.

I knew this was a good choice. I would NOT do radiation.

When we arrived home from the doctor's office, I was spent, emotionally and physically. I climbed into my nest with an ice pack and vowed to be gentle with myself. I replayed the doctor's visit in my mind, trying to relive it without fear.

I discovered something magickal in that retrospective.

I recognized just how strong and empowered I had been during this journey.

In my life I have struggled with depression more than I would like to admit, but since the diagnosis of breast cancer, my mood had actually been more positive. I concentrated on breathing and practiced mindfulness and gratitude daily. I'd been vulnerable and asked for help. Through it all, there had been a sense of grace and ease even amidst the discomfort. I was proud of myself.

After this small victory, I prepared for the follow-up with the surgeon the next day. The last time I had seen her, she told me that no one was going to want to let me out of radiation. She had been right about that.

But I had decided to turn it around. It really wasn't up to them to let me out of radiation, if you thought about it in a different way. I wasn't a child begging her parents to let her stay up past bedtime. I was a grown adult. These doctors worked for me, and it was up to me to give them permission to irradiate my breast. Sure, they had their opinions, opinions which I had been listening to since the start of this journey. But it was my opinion that counted the most. It was up to me to opt into radiation. And that wasn't going to happen.

The next morning, the nurse greeted us with a smile and asked me how I was feeling.

"Sore," I replied.

She asked if it was the incision for the lymph node giving me more trouble and when I said yes she told me most women said that.

She showed us to an exam room where I was told to change. I actually got a kick out of the outfit I got to wear in this doctor's office. Instead of the traditional paper half shirt that always gaps open to let in the draft, this "shirt" was actually a big fabric circle with a cutout in the middle your head goes through. No front, no back, no draft. And long enough to cover my tummy.

By then I'd been there enough times to realize they come in different colors. That day I got a floral pattern with orange trim. Trying to be helpful, Tom struggled to unfold the garment, claiming his fingers were too big. But I could see his hands shaking ever so slightly.

I smiled as he triumphed over the uncooperative top. He gently settled it over my head with extra care not to bump my left side.

The surgeon arrived with a smile and handed me my copy of the pathology report. That was one of the reasons I liked her. She knew how I was. We went over the same information she had given me on the phone. The margins and the lymph node were all clear.

I certainly didn't mind hearing that again.

We talked about how crazy it was to need three surgeries and the relief we both felt at getting a clear outcome. Then she asked the question I was dreading.

"When do you start radiation?"

"I'm not doing radiation," I responded.

She only slightly raised an eyebrow and asked me when I would see the radiation oncologist. I told her I was there yesterday, but I didn't elaborate on how I had lost my nerve.

This was a time for reclaiming my power.

I felt stronger that day, and when she made the case for radiation, I was ready. She gave me statistics, and I gave her feelings. She talked about recurrence, and I talked about side effects.

She couldn't convince me.

When she was comfortable that I had made my decision with the full knowledge of the risks and rewards, she asked if I was going to see the oncologist. Yes, I told her, I had an appointment in a couple weeks.

Because I had been proactive and seen the oncologist before treatment, I already knew I wasn't a candidate for chemotherapy. Even if I had been a candidate, that would have been another, "No thank you, I'll pass."

I also knew that tests indicated the DCIS was 98% estrogen receptive, and I was postmenopausal. The recommended treatment is a hormone therapy that lowers estrogen levels.

I was okay with that.

She seemed relieved and pointed out that even if I decided not to do radiation I would still be doing something preventative with the hormone therapy. My husband pointed out that the hormone therapy would be preventative for both breasts whereas radiation would only be for one.

That is not the only thing I would be doing that was preventative, I explained to her. I had been incorporating a holistic approach from the beginning, and that wasn't going to stop. I drank herbal teas and ate healthy foods, and took CBD (the non-mind-altering component of the marijuana plant).

If I didn't have any more questions for her, she told me she'd see me again in six months.

As she started out the door, she turned back and said she would write me a prescription before I go.

"Prescription for what?" I asked.

"A mammogram."

She was kidding, right?

No, not kidding. She explained that I could wait up to a month to do whole breast radiation, but before they did, they needed a mammogram. She would give me the prescription now so I didn't have to come back to get it.

She said good-bye and told me I could get dressed and pick up my prescription from the nurse on my way out.

I chuckled, keenly aware of the subtle way she had guided me back to radiation. I couldn't fault her for trying, I thought.

By the time we reached the car, I was laughing hysterically at the very thought of a mammogram. My breast was covered with multiple bruises, Steri-Strips were holding my incisions closed, it made my eyes water to raise my arm, and the slightest touch to my nipple shot searing pain throughout my body.

That boob would not be squished again any time soon!

CHAPTER 16

It was my last doctor's appointment, the oncologist. I had already met with him before the surgeries, so I knew what he was going to recommend. What I didn't know was how that appointment would test me.

I was 21 days past my third surgery, and I felt better than I had in a very long time. I was still in pain and tired easily, but I wasn't facing any more surgeries, and that was a blessing, a weight off my shoulders. I felt confident as Tom drove me to the doctor's office. One last appointment and then I would be free to heal.

Every time we pulled into that parking lot, my stomach fluttered. Two of my doctors, the mammograms and biopsies, and all the surgeries had taken place in the same building. I had to take a deep breath before I could get out of the car.

As we got off the elevator, I turned the wrong way and strode confidently toward the wrong office until Tom caught up with me and turned me around.

"Right," I said.

As we entered the correct office, I prepared myself for the fear energy I knew permeated the room. After a brief interaction with the receptionist, we found seats and waited for my name to be called.

An elderly woman with a walker sat down across from me. She pulled a bottle of water from her tote, but her arthritic hands couldn't twist off the cap. I gently slid into the seat next to her and asked if I could help. She graciously accepted, and we exchanged a few words about how difficult those little caps can be. It felt good to be of service.

As I moved back to my original seat, the woman next to me told me how she also sometimes struggled with those caps, and I agreed that some were harder than others. We engaged in idle chit chat and the next thing I knew she was pulling out a giant pill container from her purse to show me how organized she was with her medications. I heard the fear in her voice. She was doing everything she could, as if following certain rules would bring her the healing she desired. Don't we all think that way to some degree?

The nurse called my name, and we followed her back to the scale. Apparently I was feeling—and eating—better, because I gained back two of the pounds I had lost. My vitals were all good, and then she asked if I had had two lumpectomies.

"No, I actually had three," I replied with some pride.

"Wow," she said and poked around on the computer, searching for all the reports. After finishing, she told us the doctor would be in shortly and left the room.

It wasn't long before the doctor came in, introduced himself and shook our hands. He didn't remember me, but I didn't care. This was going to be short and sweet—he'd write me the prescription for the hormone therapy, and away I'd go. He introduced the young woman with him as his PA and told us she graduated just a week ago. We congratulated her, and she smiled brightly.

The doctor leaned on the exam table, shuffling through the papers in my file. "You had a lumpectomy?" he asked without looking up.

"Well, actually, three lumpectomies and a lymph node taken out," I replied.

He asked when.

I rattled off the dates, since I knew them by heart—all Mondays, remember.

He shuffled through the papers, every so often softly reading a line to himself. Still leaning on the table, he looked over his glasses at me and asked about radiation.

"I have decided not to do radiation," I said proudly.

He stopped the paper shuffling and asked why.

"I don't feel it's right for me."

I had worked through the decision after I visited the radiation oncologist, and I knew it was the right one. I assumed these were just routine questions he had to ask before he wrote the prescription. After all, he was the oncologist and had nothing to do with radiation.

I was blindsided by what happened next.

He straightened up, looked across the room at me, and said, "You're making a big mistake. You have to have radiation."

But I was not giving in so easily. "I don't want to do radiation."

"You had to have three surgeries, and you had a micro-invasion. Radiation is safe these days. There are no side effects," he said sternly.

I brought up the brittle ribs and lung damage.

He replied, dismissively, that those were minimal.

They didn't sound minimal to me.

He invited me over to the exam table. He was standing right next to me, in my space, determined to change my mind. He kept hammering away at me. At least three times he said if I were his sister he would tell me to do radiation. He listened to my heart and lungs with his stethoscope, all the while listing further reasons why I should change my mind. I felt the energy careening out of control, and I started to doubt myself. I thought I was over the scary stuff, the confrontations, the fights about radiation. This was supposed to be an in-and-out visit to get the prescription. What had happened?

I wasn't ready to give in just yet.

I asked him about the odds of recurrence. The radiation oncologist had told me, but I wanted to hear what this doctor had to say. He confirmed that if a woman doesn't do radiation, there is a 40% chance of recurrence of breast cancer.

Now it was my turn to look him straight in the eye. "Doesn't that mean that if a woman doesn't do radiation there is a 60% chance she will NOT have a recurrence?"

He didn't seem prepared for that kind of logic. Again he made the case for radiation, this time with a much more urgent approach.

I assured him I would do the hormone therapy he recommended, just not radiation, and this meant I would still be doing something preventative.

He said it would be more effective if I had radiation first.

He mistook my lack of further engagement for a concession and encouraged me to stop downstairs and make an appointment with the radiation oncologist. Her office was right there on the first floor, and I could stop in and make that appointment on my way out of the building.

He finally authorized the prescription I had come in for to begin with, and we shook hands as he left the room. The PA told me the prescription had already been transmitted to the pharmacy and showed us the way out. We got off the elevator at the first floor and walked right past the radiation oncology office without stopping.

I have a stubborn streak.

CHAPTER 17

It was autumn, finally. All my life I have been attuned to the changing seasons. Living in the desert, I had to look more closely to see the changes, but I could still feel them. The days no longer consistently reached 105 degrees. The nights got, first, into the 80s, then gradually into the 70s. We could open windows after dusk.

I was especially tuned in to the coming of autumn because the summer had been a trial. The entire summer had been consumed by the shadow of breast cancer. I danced with it, cried with it, embraced it, and tried to will it away. It took me way out of my comfort zone and brought me to my knees more than once.

And yet I am grateful.

It was a crash course in vulnerability, love, fear, gratitude, and grace.

Now what?

I knew I couldn't go back. I was not the woman I was before—I *am* not the woman I was before. But I wasn't entirely sure who I had become. I didn't want this journey with breast cancer to be without purpose. But I didn't yet know what the lesson was or how I was supposed to make a difference.

But it never hurts to take inventory. Autumn is a time to harvest the fruits of summer, reflect on our accomplishments, and prepare for the winter.

I reflected on that summer of breast cancer, and this is what I learned:

- I am important and my needs matter.
- I can be vulnerable and supported and independent and strong at the same time.
- The outpouring of love from friends, family, and community is a better pain reliever than any medication.
- One can find grace in the midst of uncertainty, and gratitude in the midst of pain.
- The world continues to function without me.

That last one was a little sobering, actually, until I thought about it more deeply and came up with this: it was freeing as well. If the world could function without me, that meant it wasn't all on me. I could let go. I could loosen my grip. I could spend more time pursuing love and joy and less time on drudgery. Of course, sometimes you have to work through the drudgery. But here's the thing about facing breast cancer. When you get through it, and you're still alive, you're grateful even for the drudgery. If nothing else, facing cancer does help to recalibrate your priorities, to appreciate all of life's canvas. I'm still learning how to do that every day.

And here's my advice to you. Don't wait until you face cancer or some other critical medical condition to figure this out. Close your laptop. Turn off the TV. Leave your phone on the desk. Then grab the nearest person by the hand and take them outside to look at the world with new eyes. Take a deep breath, feel the warmth of the sun on your cheeks or the bite of the wind. Appreciate the vastness of the sky, this gift of life. What are you doing with it? What do you want to do with it? These are worthy questions.

CHAPTER 18

At my previous oncologist visit, the doctor told me that because of the hormone therapy I needed a bone density scan and that his office would set it up and call me with an appointment. In the following ten days, I had to call the office three times, but I finally was able to set it up.

My heart dropped when the woman on the phone told me the scan would be at the Breast Center. Really? The same building where all my biopsies, surgeries, and admonishments from doctors had taken place?

I can appreciate the convenience of one-stop healthcare, but it felt like a déjà vu moment that just wouldn't quit.

Pulling into the parking lot, I couldn't help but think I hoped the doctor didn't find out I was there and try to make me do radiation again. I laughed at the idea of trying to sneak in so he didn't see me.

I found a parking spot and sat in the car taking deep breaths before I headed inside.

My heart raced a little as I walked by the radiation office on one side and the surgery center on the other to get to the elevator. I saw the sign for the oncologist's practice, and I ducked my head, then chuckled at my silliness.

I came to this appointment alone. It was just a scan; no one was going to tell me anything until they analyzed the results. I could handle this.

A bone density test uses a small dose of X-ray to measure the amount of calcium and minerals in the spine, hip, and sometimes the forearm. The higher the bone mineral content, the denser the bones. The denser the bones, the stronger they are. Bone loss was one of the risks of the hormones I was taking to lessen the chance of the breast cancer returning. Technically called an aromatase inhibitor, the medication is designed to reduce the amount of estrogen in the body. Bones are living, growing tissue. Estrogen helps build new bone. When levels are low, the existing bone breaks down faster than new bone is produced, causing holes in the spongy part of the bone. Those holes weaken the bone, which can lead to a break.

Oh, and the medication can also increase menopause symptoms. Yay! Even more hot flashes and bitchy moments.

This scan was to set the baseline before the treatment.

My body tensed as I opened the door to the Breast Center. The overwhelming pink sets me off every time, and it seemed even pinker than I remembered. It was mid-morning and the waiting room was about half full. I checked in and took a seat.

While I waited, a woman on her way out was visibly performing deep breathing exercises. I recognized that feeling of "just let me out of here." A man and woman came out of another door I knew led to the navigator's office. Their energy was pulled tightly around them, and they looked shaken.

I tried to distract myself without checking out so much I would miss my name. Waiting times in the lobby had been very short on my previous visits. I was surprised to see the room so full that day. Then I heard the woman at the desk tell a patient it was breast cancer awareness month, so they were busier than normal. That explained the wait, but I preferred to think of October as the month of Halloween and Tom's birthday. I had gotten a head start on breast cancer awareness this year.

After a long wait, my name was finally called. I followed the technician through the door to the changing room. It was just as I remembered it. She asked if I had any metal in my clothes or body. When I replied that I did not, she commended me for being prepared and told me I didn't need to change out of my clothes. I took that as a small victory—no humiliating hospital robe.

This waiting room was empty as I looked briefly out the window. It was the same window I had looked out of at the beginning of this journey and tried not to cry.

There had been many tears since that day.

But today was not a day for tears. The bone density scan was easy, just lie on the table and put my legs up on a block. It only took about fifteen minutes, and I kept my dignity intact.

I wasted no time getting back to the car and off to the rest of my day. As I drove along the building, I passed the windows I had been looking out of just a few minutes earlier. I stopped the car, and looked up at those windows.

I couldn't help but notice how different the view was from down here, the freedom of the outside looking in.

CHAPTER 19

Something was off. I didn't feel right.

I was exhausted all the time. My hips hurt so bad I couldn't lie on my side. I got waves of nausea that made me hover around the bathroom in case I had to puke. My hot flashes were worse than ever, and on and off my left hand went numb.

I'd been trying to ignore the obvious, but I couldn't any longer.

I got scared.

The symptoms had been getting progressively worse, but I had been trying to push through. The day before, I had had a full day of clients. Most of them were transformational coaching clients, but I did two massages as well. It was the first time since my surgeries that I had done more than one massage in a day.

By the end of the day, I was in real pain.

My left arm, shoulder, and breast hurt so bad I hid in the bathroom to cry. I took something for the pain and downplayed the hurt to my family. It didn't work. Apparently, I had a way of holding my left arm when that area hurt, and they noticed it right away.

After another poor night of sleep, I got up early in the morning and went in the hot tub to see if that would help. It didn't. I tried eating a small breakfast to soothe the nausea, but that didn't help either. I was so exhausted I went back to bed and lay down.

Something was definitely not right.

It was probably side effects from the medication.

Tom came in to check on me. He suggested I make an appointment with the oncologist who had prescribed the medication.

I knew he was right, but I didn't want to go see the oncologist. I remembered how discouraging it was to be told I was wrong for choosing not to do radiation. He told me that the radiation's side effects of brittle ribs and lung damage were minimal.

In my mind I had made a compromise. I wouldn't do the radiation, but I would do the hormone therapy to reduce the amount of estrogen my body made. Since the breast cancer I had had was sensitive to estrogen, this medication would in theory help prevent the breast cancer from recurring. I knew there were different options for this therapy, so it would be easy enough to switch medications.

But just the thought of making an appointment with the oncologist flooded me with fear.

I was supposed to be done with cancer.

The sign for oncology made my stomach hurt; walking through the door made me pant for breath. I kept telling myself that it was a simple visit to change medications, and there was nothing to worry about. I had made my decision about radiation, and I was sticking to it. The only thing was, I had thought I had nothing to worry about when I went for that first mammogram, either.

As soon as I stepped through the door, I felt all the old emotions flooding back. My hand shook as I signed in, and I caught that familiar scent of disinfectant and latex. The woman behind the desk didn't acknowledge me, so I found a seat to wait my turn.

The room was thick with fear, just as I remembered it. My heart filled with compassion as I looked around the room. Each person was on a personal journey with cancer. There were loved ones looking helpless, and newbies looking lost. There was a woman playing with her short spiky hair, obviously grateful for its return, while two others wearing headscarves looked on a little jealously, clearly looking forward to the time when they had that much hair again.

My eyes welled up with tears. I bent forward so no one could see, and I lightly touched Tom's arm to remind myself I was not alone. He smiled, covering my hand with his.

It was early in the morning, but the office was already behind. It was past my appointment, but there were many people in the waiting room who had arrived before me. I had no choice but to wait until they called my name.

I reminded myself to breathe.

As if to fill the vacuum, I started with the negative self-talk, to devalue myself. These people are facing "real" struggles, I told myself, and I'm here because of side effects from medication. Who cares? I should learn to live with the fatigue, nausea, joint pain, and numbness in my hand. It's no big deal. What do I expect? I don't deserve anything else.

"Now hold on," I told myself, recognizing my thought patterns for what they were—self-doubt. I quickly turned it around. My needs DO matter.

Hearing my name pulled me out of the brain chatter, and I gathered my wits as I followed the nurse through the door. She had me step on the scale, and I said hello again to those ten pounds I lost over the summer. It's okay, I told myself. I still look good. I'm still rocking it.

The nurse took my vitals and before I knew it, Tom and I were alone, waiting for the doctor. I had a moment of fear the doctor would ask me about radiation, but I knew I was past the 30-day window to have it done, so there was really nothing to talk about.

The doctor came into the room with his PA in tow and stood by the window doing his paper shuffle. "Why are you here?" he asked.

I told him the same rundown of symptoms I had told the nurse—fatigue, nausea, joint pain, and numbness in my hand.

He hadn't yet made eye contact. He told me the numbness in my arm was from surgery, and motioned for me to get up on the exam table. He listened with his stethoscope while I took two breaths and said they would call in a new prescription to the pharmacy. He shook my hand and said his PA would give me a treatment summary.

He was in and out in literally five minutes. And I was thrilled.

The PA stayed behind to finish the paperwork. I was caught off guard when she came up to me to go over it.

The papers were a cancer survivorship care plan.

The cancer history, MY journey, all documented on one piece of paper. I couldn't say anything as she went over it. She pointed out the list of all my doctors, the diagnosis, the surgeries, and the medication changes.

I didn't want to look at that paper. I took it when she offered and quickly folded it up so I couldn't see it.

Once we got to the car, I took a deep breath and began to read. There wasn't anything on the paper I didn't already know, but seeing it in such clinical black and white stirred up strong emotions.

I felt empowered when I saw the line for radiation checked "No" and written in parentheses: "Patient Declined"!

The doctor had told me to wait two weeks before taking the new medication to let the old one get completely out of my system. I was all for that! No meds for two weeks. The pharmacy won't hold a prescription that long, so we decided to stop on the way home and pick it up.

At the pharmacy, they told me the new prescription wasn't covered by insurance and cost $511 a month.

You have got to be kidding me!

They mentioned insurance might cover the medication if the doctor filled out some forms to say I really needed it.

Really?

The doctor wrote a prescription. Isn't that form enough? I would think he believes I really need the medication if he wrote the prescription.

Apparently it took more forms and more bureaucracy to get the expensive stuff.

I left without the pills, and in the two weeks I was off hormone therapy, the symptoms went away.

But eventually, I did jump through the hoops to have the prescription covered by insurance. I was feeling pretty good by the time I got approval and the second prescription was ready at the pharmacy. After just a week on the new medication, I was having worse symptoms than the first time.

After another trip to the oncologist, he gave me a prescription for the last of only three aromatase inhibitors available for my treatment. It was back to the pharmacy and more hoops to jump through with the insurance company.

Two weeks later, when I finally got the drugs, I couldn't take them. I would bring the pill to my mouth, but my hand would shake, and I just couldn't do it. Every fiber in my body was telling me "No," so I listened.

It's not what I recommend for everybody, but I never did go back on hormone therapy.

CHAPTER 20

My soul was crying out for tree time. No offense to the desert mesquite and Palo Verde trees—they have a hard-scrabble beauty of their own—but I wanted big trees. Trees that blocked the sun. Trees you can wrap your arms around and hug. Trees that sprinkle the ground with dried leaves that crinkle when you walk on them. A castle of trees, a cathedral of trees.

The nudging toward tree time started gently. Out of nowhere, I recalled a pleasant memory of walking among the peaceful northwest Redwoods. About the same time, we received a holiday card with a photo of a huge tree at the peak of its fiery fall colors. Then I had a random conversation with a friend about playing in a pile of fall leaves as a kid, how you and your friends raked them into the highest pile you could manage, then all took a running start and jumped in at the same time, screaming and laughing, spitting out the leaves that smelled of soil and tasted like dirt, all the while scattering the leaves all over the yard. Then you did it again, and again, until the leaves were so mashed up you couldn't rake them up any more.

These were all signs. Nature is a source of power for me, and my battery was running low. Each nudge caused a deeper stirring in my soul.

I preciously guarded the one day coming up in my schedule that was completely open, and declared my intention to go up north, hug some trees, and play in the water. It didn't matter if anyone else wanted to go. I was going.

Tom agreed to go along, so we packed a picnic lunch, climbed in the pickup, and headed north to Sedona. We had a particular place in mind, a little spot on the creek we know of. It isn't exactly secret, but the turnoff is unmarked, so not many people go there.

As soon as we got off the freeway, I could feel my body relax. When I stepped out of the truck, dried leaves crackled under my feet. I took a deep breath and gazed up at the towering sycamores. I was home.

Big brown leaves the size of dinner plates were strewn on the ground. I picked one up, turning it over in my hand to fully appreciate the beauty of both sides, how the network of veins flowed from the stem, how the lobes looked like the wings of a butterfly or exotic bird. A smile touched my lips as I thanked the tree for dropping this leaf. In that moment, I felt as if it had been put there just for me.

I'm sure I looked like a crazy woman running around hugging trees, throwing leaves in the air, and playing in the dirt, but it made my soul happy. The birds sang as I danced with wild abandon. Or maybe they were just laughing at me. Who knows with birds? Either way, we all seemed to be having fun.

The more I played in the woods, the more I felt like me.

Tom explored the other side of the rise, while I investigated the dry creek. Water usually flowed through the creek, but that day it was dry, and I saw rocks and ledges I had never seen before. I climbed around until I found a great place to sit on a boulder that was normally under water. I whispered gratitude for the gift of seeing that which is often unseen. I knew it was about more than the rocks. Tears came unexpectedly as I thought back on the last few months, the challenges and trials, the fear and boredom, the anger and helplessness, the sadness and, yes, joy. On that boulder, in that peaceful spot, in the midst of the cycle of life of these huge, lovely trees, the earth cleared emotional energy from my body I had been holding ever since the diagnosis.

When the tears stopped, I felt peaceful and empowered, my battery recharged.

CHAPTER 21

They say time heals all wounds.

I wasn't sure I believed that. Or maybe it just hadn't been enough time.

Even though it felt like a lifetime ago, it had only been a little more than six months since my last breast cancer surgery, and I was still a little sore. My whole left side felt weaker than the right, as if I was missing something. Oh, wait. I *was* missing something. A solid chunk of my breast and a lymph node. If I raised my arm too quickly, I felt a twinge where the lymph node had been removed. My left shoulder ached regularly, and I found myself cradling my left arm when I got tired. I'm sure some of it was in my head, but not all of it.

I was thinking about this because it was time to make an appointment for my follow-up mammogram. I hadn't had to think about doctors and diagnoses and getting put under and cut open for several blissful months. It's not that I had forgotten I had had breast cancer surgery. How could I? It was just that I didn't have to face up to it every single day. I didn't have to make momentous decisions. I didn't have that next appointment looming on my calendar and in my head. I didn't have to sit nervously in a waiting room swimming in pink anxious about the unknown. I didn't have to track and record my every pain. I didn't have to research yet another medical term or process I didn't fully understand. I didn't have to fight with doctors who wanted me to do things I wasn't prepared to do. I didn't have to make daily phone calls to doctors' offices, the insurance company, the pharmacy. I hadn't opened the medical binder in months, and in fact it was buried under other books and papers. In other words, I was living my life again.

But now I had to revisit it all and make a call to schedule that mammogram.

Mammogram. The word alone made me anxious. Isn't that how all this got started?

It was just a phone call, but the memories came flooding back.

I purposely hadn't saved the number on my phone. I didn't want to scroll through my contacts and have it pop up unexpectedly. Unfortunately, that meant I had to look in the binder to get the number.

The binder had started out neat and well organized, but as I got further along my journey and things got overwhelming, I just started stuffing papers inside of it, sometimes without reading them. As the doctors' appointments slowed down, the binder got even less attention.

With shaking hands, I dug out the binder from under all the stuff I had stacked on top of it. I had forgotten how heavy it was until I picked it up.

I knew exactly where to find the phone number. It was on the list of the doctors I had made on the first few pages. I just needed to get there. But when I opened the binder, loose papers slid out all over the desk, displaying ugly words like oncology, pathology, cancer, bone scan, medication, diagnosis, surgeon, and side effects. At least they were ugly to me, reminders of a time I was trying to put behind me. I quickly gathered up the papers and turned them face down.

I punched in the number while I still had the courage. The appointment was already overdue. I should have made it for the previous month, but I had kept putting it off.

A machine answered and put me on hold. I was probably on hold for less than a minute, but in that short time, I went through a dozen different reasons why I should just hang up. But I didn't. I decided to be an adult that day.

A friendly woman's voice came on the line and asked how she could help. I forced myself to take a deep breath and told her I needed to make an appointment for a mammogram.

I know I'm supposed to feed myself with optimism and positive mantras, but in that moment, all I could find was fear. My mind was racing with unpleasant memories, and my stomach clenched up as if I was reliving everything in that second. But I managed my fear, and let myself feel it. I'm not sure how well this was working. Feeling my fear meant that I felt, well, fearful. Was that how it was supposed to work?

After we set the appointment, the friendly woman asked if I knew where the office was located. I snorted and said, "I sure do. Been there a few times."

Tears rolled down my face after we said our good-byes and disconnected. I would be walking back into the cancer vortex in three days.

My hand trembled as I pressed the elevator button the day of the follow-up mammogram. This building held too many unpleasant memories, since it was the home of the surgery center, radiation, and oncology. This was our first time back in months.

Stepping off the elevator, my stomach fluttered with a moment of fear. I took several deep breaths to prepare myself. The office was just as I remembered it—overwhelmingly pink. I realized my hand was still shaking when I couldn't read my own name on the sign in sheet.

Sitting next to Tom, I tried not to relive all our other visits, but it wasn't easy. Nothing much had changed. The staff still wore pink uniforms, and everyone in the waiting room gave off waves of fear.

Though I have my personal reasons for not enjoying my trips to the breast health center, I do have to say that the staff and service they provide are top notch. It didn't take long for my name to be called, and I was ushered through the same door that had started this journey eight months before.

I just kept reminding myself to breathe.

Even with all the unpleasant memories, there was a small amount of comfort in knowing the routine. Place your stuff in the locker, put on a robe, wait here.

I took a seat in the waiting area and smiled softly at the other woman seated there. She smiled back nervously, and then turned to her phone for a distraction. I looked around and was disappointed to see the usual plate of cookies on the table. The herbalist in me wished they would offer healthier snacks.

I recognized the woman who came to the doorway and called my name. I followed her down the hall. She stepped aside to let me enter the room ahead of her, and I had another moment of panic. It was the same room where she had done my biopsies and inserted the guide wires before my first surgery. Had I misunderstood what this was all about? My previous mammograms had been in another room with different equipment. I was not prepared to be facing the machinery that had been a part of such unpleasant memories. I remembered my embarrassment when blood had run down the side of the machine during the biopsies, and how scared I had been before surgery.

She offered me a seat, and I took it gratefully because my knees didn't feel like they would support me right then. I forced myself to focus on answering her questions as she shuffled through my paperwork.

When I confirmed that I had been through three surgeries, she asked to see my surgical scar so she could note it in my file. After I opened my robe, she said, "I recognize that tattoo."

I nodded and told her I had been here once or twice before.

I practiced deep breathing while I stood draped over the machine, my breast flattened in various uncomfortable positions. The pain made me dizzy.

She took several pictures then told me to have a seat in the waiting area. The room was more crowded, but I didn't care. I held my breast delicately, trying to convince it to stop throbbing.

My eyes grew wide when she returned to tell me that the radiologist wanted her to take more pictures. I followed her down the hall again, my composure slipping.

The already throbbing breast was squished again. By the time she was done, I was crying from the pain. She had me sit down for a moment before releasing me to the waiting room.

I was scared.

It didn't seem like a good omen that she had to take more pictures. Had the radiologist seen something?

By the time she came back and motioned for me to follow her, I had gone through a whole range of emotions. I was determined to be strong no matter what she said.

When she looked up at me she was smiling. Everything was fine, and they would send the results to my doctor.

I didn't realize I had been holding my breath until she finished speaking and I let it out in a whoosh.

"Thank you," I said. "Thank you."

I got dressed, went out to the main waiting room, and delivered the good news to Tom. He was so relieved, he gave me a big hug, then said, "I'm sorry, I'm sorry" when he saw me wince. I waved it off. My breast was throbbing like crazy, but I didn't care.

We walked out of the building into the sun. I stopped to feel the warmth. The world had changed while I had been inside. Or at least I had. I belonged to a new club now.

I am a survivor.

CHAPTER 22

But our journey with cancer wasn't over, not by a long shot.

In the last few years, my husband Tom has been growing into the artist he has always aspired to be. He works in wood, and more and more customers are commissioning pieces, keeping him busy with orders. He always has more than one project going—cabinets, tables, wooden figures, spiritual symbols, ritual and decorative bowls, wood-burned art.

That's his happy place.

But it takes a lot of work to keep the Peaceful Spirit Enrichment Center running and Tom does most of the heavy, outdoor tasks. There are trails to rake, trees to trim, buildings to repair, rocks to move, firewood to chop, and gutters to clean. And this is just the normal maintenance for any home in New River. Whenever we have an event at the Center, Tom's workload increases. He erects the large white shade canopy, arranges the chairs and tables, lays the wood in the fire pits, creates affirmation stones, and puts out signs. He also is the one to deal with the big, unexpected repairs as well. When our septic system broke down, he was the one who did most of the digging and other labor to get it up and running again.

Every day there is something new to do at the Center.

So it didn't seem odd when Tom's shoulder started bothering him. He had been working hard for many months. He said it felt like a rib was out. He got some relief from massage—good thing he knows a good massage therapist—and visited the chiropractor regularly. Still he had a constant dull ache in the right shoulder. But he's a tough guy and he didn't complain much.

One day he came into my office from outside and said the strangest thing. "Look at my face. I'm not sweating on half my face."

It was true. He wasn't sweating on half his face. He has always sweat profusely, drenching his clothes and using bandanas or handfuls of paper towels to keep the sweat out of his eyes. I looked closely, touched the two sides of his face, and sure enough, the right side of his face was bone dry. It was as if a line had been drawn down the middle. The right side was dry, and the left was dripping. His right arm was also dry, but the rest of his body was sweating normally.

"That's odd," said the healer in me.

Meanwhile, the pain in his shoulder was getting worse, so we made an appointment with the family doctor. We felt sure he had just overworked the shoulder and the resulting inflammation was causing the pain and somehow messing with the sweat glands on that side of the body.

We both have the same general practitioner, and on the rare occasions we see her, we go together. She greeted us both warmly and asked how I was doing after breast cancer and how Tom was doing since his kidney stone. We joked about how 2016 had been a tough year for us both, but we felt better now.

Except for Tom's shoulder and face.

She examined him, checked his reflexes, and remarked on what great shape he was in. She ordered X-rays that were done in the same office and blood work to be drawn at the lab across the parking lot. Everything went smoothly, and we were home in an hour.

Tom went back to his studio to work, and I got busy on the computer, and we went on with our respective days. We were both surprised when the doctor called that evening after her office was closed. I went on the alert, remembering how unexpected doctors' calls during my ordeal were rarely good news.

She told Tom there was a shadow on his lung, and they needed a better look. She scheduled a CT scan for the next day.

We went together to the office that did his CT scan. We were understandably nervous, considering all I had gone through. This time it was Tom's turn to strip down and dress in the unflattering hospital gown and get taken into the room by himself for the procedure. I quickly realized that being on this side of the door wasn't easy either. I paced around the waiting room more for Tom than I ever did for myself.

Finally, Tom returned, dressed in his own clothes, and I couldn't help asking, "How'd it go?"

"Nothing to it," he said. "They just took pictures."

"Right," I said, and we returned home.

The doctor called a few hours after the scan. Uh-oh. Another unexpected call from a doctor. She told us they had found what looked like a Pancoast tumor on his right lung. We felt better when she told us she had seen valley fever that looked just like this.

Since Tom didn't have any lung symptoms such as coughing or shortness of breath, valley fever seemed reasonable, but there was the possibility it could be something else.

I knew it was a mistake, but I googled Pancoast tumor anyway. I didn't like what I read. On WebMD it stated: "Pancoast Tumor is a type of lung cancer that forms at the very top of the lung." What? Lung cancer? Aren't we jumping ahead here? I didn't share this information with Tom. I figured we would know for sure soon enough.

While we were setting up all the different diagnostic appointments, Tom developed an alarming new symptom. Every evening sometime between five and eight, Tom doubled up in excruciating pain. It lasted only about 20 minutes, but it was intense. It broke my heart to see him in such pain.

After two MRIs, a visit to a lung doctor, several calls between schedulers and doctors pulling strings, Tom was scheduled for a biopsy just 12 days after the first X-ray.

He was his usual charming self with the prep nurse. It was early in the day, and he was feeling good. The doctor who would be doing the biopsy was friendly and explained everything they were going to do.

I stayed with Tom until they wheeled him down the hall. He looked so vulnerable in that ugly hospital gown. When he rounded the corner, and I couldn't see him anymore, I let myself cry.

It went more quickly than I expected, and he was in recovery 40 minutes later. The tears had dried, and I was back in protector mode. He had to have two chest X-rays with no complications over the next three hours before they would let him leave.

He did well.

It was 5:14 pm the next day when his doctor called. She called both our cell phones but we missed the calls because our ringers had been turned down. It was 5:21 when I saw the missed call. I immediately called her office. It had to be the biopsy results.

An answering machine picked up and told me the office was closed but the urgent care center was still open. The doctor and urgent care are both in the same office and they share a reception desk and staff. I chose the option for the urgent care side in the hopes that I could get a live person to put me through to the doctor side.

I didn't want another sleepless night.

A woman answered the phone. I explained our plight and she agreed to see if the doctor's assistant was still in the office. I thanked her and tried to breathe while I waited on hold.

She came back and told me the assistant was still there and she would transfer my call to her. I relaxed a little as the phone rang to that extension.

The answering machine picked up.

Nooooo!

I hung up and dialed the main number again. No matter what extension I dialed this time, I got an answering machine. I frantically dialed over and over trying to get a live person. According to my phone log I called 14 times in 6 minutes, each time getting that damn answering machine.

Finally, I looked at Tom and said, "Let's get in the truck and go down there right now." I knew it was a long shot, but the office was only ten minutes away, and this was important. By now it was 5:35 and I wasn't sure anyone would still be there, but it was worth a try.

When we arrived I told the woman at the reception desk what had happened. She thought everyone from the doctor's office had left, but she agreed to go back and look. She came out and told us that the medical assistant had already left, but believe it or not the doctor was still there and would see us.

Suddenly my feet felt like lead, and I balked. Tom took me by the hand and guided me through the door to meet with the doctor. He smiled to ease my fear, but I wasn't buying it. I could see the worry in his eyes.

The doctor shook our hands and offered us a seat in her office. I apologized for the unconventional way we had arrived after hours, but she didn't mind. She told us that she had in fact called us with the biopsy results.

The biopsy showed that the tumor on Tom's lung was cancer.

CHAPTER 23

Hearing that Tom had lung cancer was more devastating to me than my own diagnosis for breast cancer. I can see myself as broken, or at least in need of healing, but not him. He's invincible. He's strong, smart, kind, funny, creative, and caring. He's my world. He's my hero. He's my husband. He's my soul mate, the love of my life.

Which is why, at Tom's diagnosis, I felt like I had been punched in the stomach. And the face. And everywhere else, as if I had been worked over in a boxing gym.

He handled it with his usual charm, even to the point of consoling the doctor when she delivered the news.

The week after went by in a blur. There were eight medical visits in five days. Tom's veins were poked six times, and he was sedated, magnetized, and x-rayed, and had targets placed on his torso. He was injected with radioactive contrast twice. We laughed that he would soon be glowing in the dark.

Tom was referred to the same oncologist I had seen, which gave me another stomach churning moment. The doctor never let on if he remembered me or not. And though he hadn't been a good fit for me, he was great as Tom's doctor.

We liked his radiation doctor as well, a different doctor than I had seen. She took the time to explain all the images and her treatment plan. She told us that Tom needed to see a surgeon very soon to determine whether the tumor was operable. The surgeon's assessment would also determine the dose of radiation.

The energy and urgency of the whole thing was overwhelming. Our emotions ran from hopeful to mournful and back again like waves on a beach.

It was a Friday morning and our second visit to the oncologist that week. I was exhausted from worrying too much and sleeping too little. Tom looked tired, too, but he still had a smile for the nurse as she raised an eyebrow over his elevated blood pressure.

The doctor arrived with test results in hand. He got straight to the point. Stage 3 non-small cell carcinoma.

My heart sank. Stage 3.

We talked about a treatment plan—surgery, if the cancer hadn't spread too far, then radiation and chemotherapy. He explained everything thoroughly, and we were given handouts to digest at home. His smile seemed genuine when he said the cancer was treatable.

He made sure we didn't have any more questions before shaking our hands goodbye and leaving us with his assistant. She gave us the prescriptions for fentanyl patches, oxycodone, and two anti-nausea medications, and led us out into the hall to show us around.

I hadn't prepared myself to see the chemotherapy room. I knew what one looked like, since I had supported others through this part of their journey. But this time it was for Tom.

We rounded the corner, and there was a room full of recliners with IV poles standing neatly next to them. Fortunately, the room was empty because I stopped suddenly in my tracks and drew an audible breath.

Immediately, Tom was there to steady me. Did I mention he was superman?

I backed quickly out of the room and started to cry. Our guide located some tissues and then was briefly called away. I was grateful for the moment to compose myself.

We left the office with a sigh of relief that it was the last visit at the end of a very long week. We would have a couple days off before the next round.

With any major health issue, there is the process of telling your tribe. Tom knew right away that he wanted to keep his three kids up to date. He asked me to make the first calls. I called each one individually and put them on speakerphone with him sitting beside me. His eyes welled up with tears when he heard the emotion in each of their voices.

He couldn't talk at the beginning of the call but eventually he would get control of his tears and let them know he was on the line. He talked with each of them for a long while, and they all shared how much they loved each other. You could tell his heart was full when they were done.

Those two days went by fast, and Monday we were back at the doctor's office. Referrals were made, schedules were rearranged, and last-minute plans changed to get Tom an appointment with a surgeon. Knowing we had been squeezed in gave us a little more patience for the 75-minute wait.

We immediately liked the surgeon, he is a specialist in lung transplants, chief surgeon at the hospital, and a professor. He seemed very qualified. We also liked the fact that this practice used a program to record the visits and make them available online. There is so much information given in an appointment like that. It is helpful to go back and listen to it again.

The surgeon explained that he would biopsy the lymph nodes near the tumor to see if they had cancer in them. If they were infected, then there was no chance of surgery. Surgery was what we wanted at this point. Surgically removing the tumor meant a better chance of survival.

The biopsy would be outpatient surgery under general anesthesia. The surgeon explained that he would first go down the throat with a flexible scope to do a needle biopsy. If he found cancer, he would stop. If he didn't find cancer but was still suspicious, he would cut a hole at the base of Tom's throat and use a metal tube to get bigger samples of the lymph nodes.

I hugged Tom tightly before they wheeled him away for the biopsy. I could feel him shaking slightly, but I didn't want to ask whether he was cold or scared.

The waiting room at the hospital was not well supplied. There was only coffee, no water, and not a box of tissues to be seen. Fortunately, I had come prepared with water, snacks, reserve tissues, and moral support.

Being the stubborn person I am, I initially resisted my girlfriend's request to come to the hospital with us. Looking back now, I am grateful she didn't listen to me.

The surgeon came out after the flexible scope and told us the lymph nodes he got were clean, but he had seen something that made him suspicious, so he was going ahead with the incision and bigger samples. He would come back and let us know when he was done.

It was an even longer wait this time. The surgeon called us out into the hall and gave us the news. There was cancer in the lymph nodes. It had metastasized.

I stood there and looked at him in disbelief. Take it back, I wanted to say. I wanted to go get Tom, go home, and pretend this never happened.

I wanted the hole in my chest to stop hurting.

But the surgeon kept talking, and I made myself pay attention. Surgery was no longer an option because it wouldn't increase Tom's chances of survival. He didn't sugarcoat the outcomes for a Stage 3 Pancoast tumor.

My girlfriend and I both kept asking the same questions in different ways, hoping to get different answers. The doctor was patient with us as we wiped away tears and tried to make sense of it all. He told us that a nurse would take us to see Tom in recovery.

It was almost two hours before they called us to see him. We went through boxes of tissues and countless emotions. I kept telling myself to get it together, but every time I thought about telling him what the doctor said, I cried harder.

I didn't expect him to be fully awake and dressed when we saw him in recovery. He had a two- by three-inch white bandage at the base of his throat and was visibly in pain. I kissed him and tried to keep my emotions in check.

There was a flurry of activity around him. One nurse was trying to do his discharge papers, and another was taking out his IV and disconnecting him from the monitors. The nurse told my girlfriend where to park the car and wait for them to bring Tom down in a wheelchair.

The busyness around him had kept me from telling him what the doctor said. The nurse told me she had just given him something for pain, and then she was gone.

Suddenly we were alone and it was quiet. Tom had his head down and was holding his throat against the pain. When he realized it had quieted down, he looked up and saw me standing there.

His eyes filled with tears and his voice was unsure when he let me know the doctor had told him the cancer was in the lymph nodes. I couldn't hold it together any longer and started to cry as I went to his side and gingerly hugged him. He whispered quietly in my ear, "Don't worry. I'll still take care of you."

I didn't know my heart could hurt that much.

CHAPTER 24

Tom stood looking in the bathroom mirror. "Draw a smiley face on it," he said. He was referring to the white gauze bandage at the base of his throat. He thought it would be funny to have a smiley face peeking out of his shirt collar.

I didn't want to hurt him, so I didn't get right to it.

He was still heavily medicated but that didn't stop him from drawing it himself by looking in the mirror. It may not have been a work of art, but it eased the tension.

We had experienced so much raw emotion since returning from the hospital. We were talking about things we didn't even want to think about. It was tough.

I am usually the crier of the family and I did an excellent job of it, but mine weren't the only wet eyes in the house.

The smiley face had a way of making us laugh through the tears.

Tom's biopsy surgery had been the Friday before a long weekend. We had three days without appointments. He was scheduled to begin radiation and chemotherapy the next Tuesday.

Given my experience, we wondered if that was the right approach.

Then the pain got intense. The week before, Tom had been put on a pain patch, which he still had on after surgery, according to one of the nurses. As the anesthesia wore off, however, his pain increased. Even though he was taking pills for breakthrough pain, it got so bad I thought we would have to take him to the emergency room.

Finally, we took his shirt off to check the patch. It wasn't there! Apparently, it had fallen off or been removed at the hospital. A few days later he would get a new patch, with double the dosage just to keep up with the pain. And even that didn't always work.

It was scary to think how much pain that medication was masking.

Tom slept a lot, and I watched him like a hawk. I warned him I would be overprotective and we would just have to work through it because I wasn't going to stop.

That weekend I became more emotionally exhausted than I have ever been in my life. So much so that it affected me physically.

It was supposed to be a quick trip to the grocery store and one other stop, a route that I had driven hundreds of times. I hesitated to leave Tom, but he was in good hands at home and I needed the distraction.

I had a short list for the grocery store and quickly picked up everything we needed. I was headed for the checkout when I landed in the Halloween aisle. I couldn't help but stop and browse. I picked up a tiny spooky house and my thoughts went to what I would have Tom do with it for the fairy garden—build a base, for one thing, to make sure it was sturdy.

There was a catch in my throat when I realized that my strong, vital, super Tom wouldn't be doing much for a while. I started to shake. Tears welled in my eyes. I set the item down as if it had burst into flames and made a beeline for the self-checkout. I kept my head down so no one could see me falling apart.

I got in my car and headed for the other stop, a quick in and out. I went through the town of Anthem on a road I know well, turned left on another road I know well, and suddenly I was lost. I could not remember where the store was, and at that moment I had no clue where I was, either. I went completely blank. I tried desperately to get my brain to function. I tried to think my way through it. I rubbed my temples and my face. I pounded on the steering wheel. Nothing worked.

I pulled into a parking lot, and sat there, engine running. I'm pretty sure I went catatonic, but for how long, I don't really know. Not too long. I jerked awake as if from a bad dream, recognized where I was, skipped my other errand, and drove home very, very carefully, staying right at the speed limit and gripping the steering wheel as if it were a lifeline.

This whole experience scared me more than a little.

I got home safely. With deep breathing and meditation, I slowly got a better grip on my emotions. I wouldn't do anyone any good, least of all Tom, if I checked out whenever things got tough. There were many more difficult conversations to come, but I felt more grounded and in control.

Partly because of the enormous amount of pain, Tom decided that radiation was right for him. It would shrink the tumor and take pressure off the nerves, relieving pain and restoring the ability to sweat on his right side. At least that was the hope.

He still wasn't sure about chemotherapy.

The first radiation treatment was quick and easy. Since it was only a short ride to the oncology office from the radiation center, we decided to try to get in to see the oncologist even though we didn't have an appointment. Tom had new questions now that the surgeon had confirmed the cancer had spread to the adjoining lymph nodes. We were both quiet in the car on the drive over.

Tom was his usual charming self when he told the receptionist he wasn't supposed to see the doctor that day but he had more questions before he started treatment and could they possibly squeeze him in. Even with the charm, his request threw everything off.

The phlebotomist came to get him, and we said no, he wanted to see the doctor. We waited for another hour before they figured out what we needed and how they could accommodate us. To be honest, neither of us was in a hurry. We didn't want to hear more bad news.

Finally, there was a flurry of activity. They called him in, and then told us to sit on the bench and wait. That was where the doctor found us. He had a genuine look of concern on his face and asked what was wrong. Tom explained about the surgeon's findings and wanted to know about his quality of life.

The doctor looked him square in the eye and said, "Even though surgery isn't an option, I believe we can cure this with chemo and radiation."

Cure? Yes!

It wouldn't be easy, the doctor explained. The treatments were long and grueling, but before this, Tom had been healthy and active, and he was committed to beating this. These would all work in his favor.

As Tom sat in his first chemo treatment that afternoon, the physician's assistant brought us a folder with more paperwork. After she walked away, I opened the folder and my eyes again filled with tears. I leaned over to Tom with one of the papers and pointed to the words on the page:

Therapy Goal: Cure.

Prognosis: Good.

CHAPTER 25

I had planned this trip months before Tom's diagnosis. It was the annual meeting of an international organization called Gather the Women.

Because of my work with women's empowerment and the monthly circles held at the Peaceful Spirit Enrichment Center, Gather the Women had invited me to join and serve as a regional coordinator back in the spring.

Each month since joining the group, I had participated in the virtual circle of regional coordinators and was excited to meet them in person.

When Tom's treatment plan was outlined, I considered cancelling the trip. There were just too many unknowns. Of all the voices that encouraged me to go, Tom's was the most convincing.

I wasn't sure I was going until a week before the scheduled departure. I had tried to keep my excitement limited and my expectations low, a coping mechanism I developed during my battles with low self-esteem.

Tom was doing well and a plan was in place to support him. I truly believed he would be okay while I was gone.

I let myself get excited.

The gathering was in Colorado, about 60 miles north of Denver, at a place called Peaceful Valley. A shuttle would take me from the airport to the gathering, and I would be staying there for three and a half days. In the woods! In nature! And the leaves would be changing for Fall! I was long overdue for another tree hug and could already feel my soul dancing in the forest.

About the time I allowed myself to get excited, one of my very dear friends experienced a life shattering event. Our circle of friends rallied around her for support. The depth of her pain reminded me to put aside my own stuff to help her get through this terrible time.

As a result, I stayed up very late the night before my flight to Denver. I had to be at the airport the next morning at 6:30, but I didn't finish packing until after midnight. My mind was racing so much I didn't sleep well and still felt exhausted when the alarm went off at 4:30. But the thought of dancing in the trees by the afternoon had me out of bed in a flash and ready to go without a hitch. If I had forgotten to pack anything, I didn't care.

After a half-hearted argument, Tom ended up driving me. We arrived at the airport right on time. I took several deep breaths to keep my composure as we said our goodbyes on the curb.

There was no line at security, and my gate was easy to find. I found an open chair and sat down with an audible sigh, exhausted but on my way. We boarded the plane on time, heard the proper announcements, and felt ourselves being pushed away from the gate. The plane stopped moving and we sat a few minutes before the captain came on the speaker and told us there was a fuel leak in one of the engines.

That didn't sound good.

After an hour and 45 minutes, they decided it couldn't be fixed while we were all still on the plane, so we rolled back to the gate, gathered up our carry-ons, and exited. They told us it was going to be a while, brought us sandwiches, chips, soda, and water and asked for our patience.

Four hours after our original departure time, they loaded us back on the same plane. It was very hot onboard. The flight attendant told us the crew was coming over from another flight, and as soon as the captain arrived he would turn on the A/C. Finally, the pilots arrived, the airplane started to cool down, and the flight attendants were told to prepare. I took a deep breath and hoped I could get a little sleep despite the kid behind me kicking my seat. I was too exhausted to complain.

Again, we pushed back from the gate…and again we stopped.

It didn't take long for the pilot to come on the speaker and tell us there was still a fuel leak in the engine and the plane would have to be taken out of service. There was a collective groan from the passengers.

By the time we all deboarded the plane, they were back with the sandwiches but they still couldn't tell us when we would get to Denver. I was starting to panic a little. I called the shuttle company and changed my reservation for the third time. The lady was very nice, but the shuttles were mostly sold out, and it was hard to move me around.

And still we waited.

Finally, they announced another plane would be coming in and we could use it to get to Denver. There was just one problem. It was too late for me. I couldn't make the shuttle in Denver. I kept frantically doing the math in my head, but no matter what I tried, I couldn't make it work. I was exhausted, overwhelmed, disappointed, and sad. I cried.

It was so hard to call Tom and say the words, "Come and get me."

By the time he met me at the curb I was having a meltdown. His energy was so loving and it was obvious how bad he felt for me. But I was so disengaged that all I could do was get in the truck and cry.

I cried off and on all the way home. Every time I looked out the window and saw desert mountains, my eyes welled up because I was supposed to be looking at trees. I was crying over more than just the missed trip, of course. We had had such a tough year, and experienced so many sad things. They all caught up with me that day.

When I got home, I went straight to bed. It had been a long time since I had felt so exhausted emotionally, physically, and mentally.

I cried myself to sleep.

It was 10:30 at night when I stirred out of bed. The house was dark and quiet, everyone else was sleeping. I had a pounding headache from crying so much and was feeling extremely sorry for myself.

Without thinking, I found myself in the Labyrinth. As I walked to the center, I acknowledged the anger, pain, and frustration I was feeling. By acknowledged I meant I was pissed off and looking for something to blame. A part of me still felt the Universe had let me down on this one. I wanted to go on that trip! I needed to go! I deserved to go!

At the center of the Labyrinth, I found some peace. I took responsibility, and when I did, the energy shifted. It had been up to me, and ultimately, I chose not to go. The airplane's difficulties hadn't helped, but I could have figured something else out on the other end. A car rental. A bus. A shuttle the next day. I took a deep breath and said to myself, "Yes, this sucks. But it happened and here I am. Let's get on with it."

When I got back to the bedroom, I found Tom restless and unsettled. It was obvious he was worried about me, but there seemed to be more to it.

Things got progressively worse.

His pain was intense. He had a nose bleed, sweats, chills, nausea, trouble swallowing, and the shakes. He threw the covers on and off as his temperature jumped around. At one point, his speech was so garbled I couldn't make sense of his words.

I put a new pain patch on his back, gave him nausea pills, herbal tea, and the breakthrough pain pills. My heart ached as I worked on a sudden muscle spasm in his neck. I considered the ER.

All night he floated in and out. It was the scariest night we had since he started treatment.

Just before dawn, the crisis broke. We got his pain under control, his temperature stabilized, and he could think and speak again. He looked at me with love in his eyes and said, "I couldn't have gotten through this night without you."

I think he was right.

He finally fell into a restful sleep, and I pulled the covers up around him. I closed the blinds to keep the room dark and help him stay asleep. I went around the house turning off lights and picking up after the long night.

The sun was just peaking over the top of the mountains when I stopped at the window to watch it rise in its red-orange splendor. I was still exhausted, but relieved and elated. We had made it through the night. Today was a new day.

I stood there thinking about what Tom had said. That's when I knew in my heart that was the plan all along—I was supposed to be there to get him through the night. There had been times when his only way through the pain was the sound of my voice. If I hadn't been there, who knows what might have happened.

I would love to tell you that I had some great insight and saw the Universe's plan for me in crystal clarity out the window that morning.

But I didn't.

Well, maybe a small insight. I had needed to be there that night for Tom.

I went back to bed and slept lightly until Tom got up feeling better. He grew stronger throughout the day.

Sure, I was disappointed I didn't get to go on the trip, but I was more grateful I had gotten to stay.

CHAPTER 26

The familiar chirp of my cellphone signaled a text message. For a minute the message didn't make sense. It was from the scheduling department of Arizona Oncology.

"Reply YES to confirm your family's 5 appts. starting at 11:00 am."

Both Tom and I had appointments the same day. We would both see the doctor and have blood drawn, then he would have a chemo treatment. I understood how they got to five appointments, but it was a shock to see it on the screen.

Then it hit me. They have an automatic program that can notify you when multiple family members have multiple appointments.

Think about that for a minute. That means it is so common for multiple family members to have multiple appointments that it is a normal part of the program.

We were not unique, Tom and I. Other families were going through this, too.

My stomach hurt as I stared at the screen. This would be the first time I had seen the oncologist for a breast cancer follow-up in six months. In all Tom's appointments, the oncologist had never let on if he remembered me or not.

I was going to find out.

We came as a set that day, Tom and I both filling out our paperwork at the same time, sitting side by side to get our blood drawn, standing together at the scale.

Oh hell no. Not at the scale!

I only keep one secret from Tom, and that's my weight.

After the scale, we reunited in the exam room. Blood pressures, temperatures, and oxygen rates were entered for each of us, and then we were left together to wait for the doctor.

How did this happen? Both of us being treated by the same cancer doctor? This was not the reality I had meant to create.

It turned out the doctor did remember me and my three surgeries and the three medications and their side effects.

He was stumped when I told him about the excruciating pain in my breast and shoulder that had sent me to the emergency room 12 days earlier. The ER doc had given me two shots of morphine that didn't touch the pain, and when they gave me a shot of valium I became unresponsive. Fortunately, oxygen brought me around. They never did figure out why I was in pain.

Since I was already scheduled for a bilateral mammogram in a few days, he examined me and said let's wait for the results.

Next was Tom's turn. The doctor asked how he was feeling and listened to his lungs. The lungs sounded good. Tom tried to lighten the mood with a chuckle when he admitted that some things were starting to get difficult. Small things, like swallowing and eating.

After the doctor, it was time for Tom's chemo treatment. Even though I wasn't getting treatment, we still went as a set into the infusion room. He got the big chair, and I pulled up a small one beside him and held his hand.

For the next few hours, we tried to act like this wasn't crazy, us sitting together in the infusion room, chatting about anything and everything—our twisted version of quality time.

CHAPTER 27

There were several days of mail in the box when I opened it. So many things had been going on, getting the mail just wasn't on the priority list. Those days the mail didn't bring many good things anyway: besides the usual ads addressed to Current Resident, doctors' bills and EOBs from insurance companies made up the bulk of it.

I skimmed through the pile as I walked back to the truck. A white envelope stood out from the others. It had my name on it, and appeared to be from the Breast Center. I thought I knew what it was, but the return address made me queasy.

I stuffed the mail in one of the grocery bags in the front seat of the truck. But that white envelope stuck out just enough to taunt me.

As I walked through the door, Tom was lying on the couch looking very weak and pale. We both knew that normally he would have met me at the car and carried everything in himself. My heart skipped a beat seeing him there. The past two months had been hard on him. He made a move to get up to help me, but I smiled and said I could manage.

With the groceries safely on the counter, I took out the mail and looked around for the letter opener. Even though I knew what the letter should say, my hand was shaking a little as I unfolded it and skimmed the paragraph.

I saw what I was looking for just as Tom got up from the couch. I quickly put the letter back in the envelope and set it down with the rest of the mail. I thought now wasn't the time to share it.

There was an all too familiar look of pain on his face. He had endured six weeks of radiation with a good spirit and open heart, but his body was paying the price. The outward signs of radiation were mild compared to what was going on inside.

It wasn't until almost the end of the 30 treatments that his right collarbone got a burn about the size of my little finger across the top of it. We were hoping he would not have any visible burns, so it seemed a less than optimal outcome to us, but to the doctor it was remarkable that that was all the burning he had.

All through treatment his radiation doctor had commented on how wonderful his skin looked and how little damage he had. At his fifth weekly visit, she finally asked what we were using on his skin that kept it looking so good.

Tom was happy to tell her about the all-natural Herbal Healing Salve that I make and sell. We had been using it on the burn area since his very first treatment. After questioning me about the ingredients, frequency of use, and how it was made, she asked if she could have a sample. I dropped off a sample the next day and at Tom's next visit she told me she had already recommended it to one of her patients.

But his visible burn was not the source of his pain today; it was the damage inside. Tom's throat was burned so badly swallowing was nearly impossible. Even water hurt going down. He knew he needed to eat to keep up his strength, but after just a few bites he would be in so much pain it brought tears to his eyes.

That day was the first day in six and a half weeks he hadn't had a radiation or chemo treatment. It was cause for celebration, but he was feeling so terrible that a weak woo-hoo was all he could muster.

His birthday was just a few days later, and he still felt miserable. He received a birthday cake, but his throat still wasn't working, so he couldn't eat it. The last few weeks had been brutal, and he was struggling. But even when he felt his worst he kept his sense of grace and compassion for others.

He had a particularly bad night and was feeling pretty low the next morning. Even though he couldn't eat, he pulled out the chair for me to sit down beside him while I ate my breakfast.

Our dining table is the catch-all for everything. Sometimes we have to move piles to make room to eat, and this morning was one of those. Tom moved a pile of mail to make room for my food, and the white envelope fell to the floor.

He picked up the envelope, and when he saw my name on it, he asked what it was.

"Just my latest test results," I said as I sat down to eat.

It felt wrong to be eating in front of him when his throat was so sore so I got quiet and focused on my food. I didn't see him pull the letter out of the envelope.

When I looked up, he was reading the letter and crying. "Why didn't you show me this?" he asked.

"You already knew everything was okay," I told him.

His voice cracked, "I know, but this is different. Seeing it in writing gives me hope."

The letter read:

> *We wish to inform you that there is no evidence of cancer on your recent mammogram examination.*

Finally some good news.

CHAPTER 28

I heard Tom sit up on the edge of the bed. "Are you all right?" I asked softly, trying not to startle him in the dark.

"I can't sleep, I'm shaking again," he replied.

The last time he had the shakes was when he stepped down the dosage on his pain patch and went through withdrawal. Every time he tried to fall asleep he would get the shakes so bad it would bounce him awake. He couldn't sleep or even relax for several days. Finally, he adjusted to the new dosage, but it was hard getting there.

He was a hippie from the sixties and had never become addicted to opioids, but now that he was *in* his sixties, the pharmaceutical industry had managed it in two months.

That night, though, it seemed that he simply might have been overtired and his nervous system was having trouble turning off. He took some herbal remedies and was eventually able to fall back to sleep. I whispered a quiet thank you in the darkness when I heard him gently snoring.

Now I was the one who couldn't sleep. My body was willing, but my brain had started to worry.

At Tom's last chemo appointment, the receptionist had presented us with an unexpected bill for $121. I tried to hide my panic. A sign on the desk read *All money due must be paid at the time of your appointment.* I could see the worry in Tom's eyes; he didn't want to miss a treatment.

I handed her my debit card even though I knew there wasn't that much in the checking account. I prayed that overdraft protection would cover it. When she handed me the receipt to sign, I breathed a sigh of relief. It cost me in bank fees, but Tom received his treatment that day.

I've heard that when you become an enlightened being, you don't worry about money—but I'm not there yet. Not many of us are.

My face stretched into a yawn and I snuggled under the covers. The next day was Thanksgiving, and I didn't have to get up early. I was looking forward to a low key, easy day as I finally drifted back to sleep.

The sun was up by the time I awoke. I took my time and did some stretching before getting out of bed. The kettle was already heating water for tea when I got to the kitchen, and the fake fireplace was on to give the illusion of a winter's day. It was forecast to be a record setting 89 degrees that day.

Even though it was going to be a hot Thanksgiving, we were all in a good mood and looking forward to the holiday. In the last week, Tom's appetite had returned and he was excited about the day's menu: turkey, gluten-free dressing, mashed potatoes, green beans, corn, cranberry sauce, and, of course, pumpkin pie. I smiled when he sang the silly song from *Michael*, the movie in which John Travolta plays an angel: "Pie, pie, me oh my. I love pie."

I decided to take a quick shower before breakfast. Even though it was a scaled back menu, I was excited about cooking. It made things seem normal.

For just a little while I didn't want to think about cancer, doctors' appointments, or side effects. I wanted to watch the Macy's parade on TV while I made a meal that would put us all in a food coma for the afternoon.

The bathroom door opened not long after I got in the shower. Tom asked if the water was backing up on me because he could hear the toilets percolating. As if on cue, the water started to rise in the shower. I rushed to rinse the shampoo out of my hair and get out before water started spilling onto the floor.

Even after spending thousands of dollars on a new leach line, we were still having problems with our septic system. The last time he came out, the plumber had run a camera through the line and told us that the line from the house to the septic tank was clogged with roots and would have to be replaced.

That line runs through the laundry room under six inches of concrete. He told us how much the repair would cost, and my heart sank.

He was very kind when we told him we couldn't afford the repairs. He told us to try root killer to keep the line clear, but even if that worked now, at some point, we would have no choice except to fix it.

The root killer didn't work.

This was a snag in our Thanksgiving plans, but we had been down this road before and knew what to do. Tom grabbed the plunger and started working. He could usually get it moving.

But not today.

He tried all the tricks, but nothing worked. He got bigger tools. Still nothing.

The harder he tried, the more frustrated he became. In just the last few days, he had started to feel stronger and more like himself. But this was taking a toll. This was the most strenuous physical activity he had done since starting treatment. He had the desire and the know-how, but his body wasn't up to it. The half of his face that could sweat was doing so profusely, and he couldn't catch his breath. I wasn't helping the situation by standing at the bathroom door telling him to stop before he hurt himself. It was breaking my heart to see him down on the floor doubled over trying to breathe. He had fought so gallantly to this point in his illness, I didn't want him to keel over plunging the toilet.

When he finally gave up two hours later, I considered it a victory.

But I had been too wrapped up in my own fear to realize how important this had been for him. There was sadness and anger in his eyes, and he didn't want to talk to me as he stormed off to his studio.

There's a lesson here for caretakers of those who are ill, whether short- or long-term. Dignity. Allow—and nurture—the dignity of those you are caring for in whatever form it takes. For Tom, it was trying to fix the toilet. For others it might be going to the bathroom on their own or cooking their own meal. Now I'm not saying we should let them put themselves or anyone else in danger. As with many things in life, it's about tone and attitude. We can say, "Let me help you," in a way that is loving and supportive. Or we can say it with a tone of resentment and even contempt. Patience comes in handy in these cases.

This insight came to me later, as insights often do. At that moment, my emotions were running high, and I slammed around the house gathering up the makings for pumpkin pie. We couldn't use any water in the house, so everything would have to be carried over to the retreat center—Sunshine House—to cook.

Once the pie was in the oven, I sat down and cried. Even on this day of all days—the one day we were going to forget about everything and just be, just let it all go—the universe rose up and bit us in the ass. Why couldn't we have one day—just one day—where we didn't have to worry about anything? Everything seemed out of control and I was so damn tired of worrying about money. We had great abundance in our lives, but at that moment, not in our bank accounts. That's the thing about owning your own business. You don't get paid sick leave. There's no coasting while you recover. There's no one else to carry you. It's all on you, and when you're not there, nothing gets done and no money comes in.

But I didn't want to be sad that day. I made a conscious effort to pull myself back from crazy town. It helped that the pie's spicy incense was wafting through the house.

When the pie was done, I texted a picture of it to Tom as a peace offering. We gathered at Sunshine House and started working things out. We shared our feelings and a few more tears, but we got back on track. I told Tom how scared I was and how I didn't want to lose him. Tom told me how scared he was and how helpless he felt not being able to do what he had always done—take care of the Center; take care of me. We both agreed that we had no idea how we were going to pay for all this—the treatments and the septic tank. And then we both agreed we would not worry about it any longer on that of all days.

It turned out to be an adventure having our Thanksgiving at Sunshine House. We figured out how to stream video on the smart TV so we could watch a funny movie while we ate our dinner. It may not have been the day we planned, but when I looked around the table all I saw was love looking back at me.

We had to go through some crap to get there—literally, in this case—but the day turned out pretty well, and we got to enjoy our food coma after all.

CHAPTER 29

We were sitting in the waiting room again, but this time was different; this was the last one—this was the last chemo treatment in Tom's regimen.

I looked over at Tom and could see the toll the treatments had taken on him. His face was thin, and he looked tired. He got winded easily, and there were new worry lines on his forehead. His pants were baggy, and his leather belt had so many new holes it looked like a sieve.

But he still didn't look like a cancer patient.

His eyes sparkled when he was feeling good, and even when he didn't feel good, he still mustered a smile for those around him. And his hair. He still had it. It was whiter and thinner than it had been, but with all the radiation and all the chemo, he never lost it. The doctor told him that he would probably lose his hair from the last two mega doses. The doc was wrong.

He smiled when he caught me looking at him. He had started to feel stronger in the previous few days and my heart hurt at the thought of him going through those chemo after-effects again. Those were long, ugly days that took us to the brink of despair.

But that was the good thing—he *had* been feeling stronger, so we knew he could get through this last one.

I looked around and allowed myself to feel the energy in the room. As always, the room was heavy with fear and anxiety. Everyone in the room either had cancer or cared deeply about someone who had cancer. Normally, I tried to shield myself from the energy in the room because it can be overwhelming.

It felt as if I had been coming here forever. First as a patient, now as a caregiver. The same artwork hung on the wall and the giant coffee machine in the corner still groaned loudly. The one time the place had looked different had been on Halloween, when many of the staff had dressed in costumes. Everyone in the room laughed when the infusion nurse came out dressed as Darth Vader and called a patient's name. The phlebotomists were dressed as vampires, and there was a pumpkin decorating contest.

Hard to believe it was after Thanksgiving already. Time seemed all scrambled up.

After his blood draw, Tom came back to the waiting room. I touched the bandage on his arm and commented on how well his veins were holding up. He had wanted to avoid a port, so he had worked hard to stay hydrated. It had taken a great deal of willpower to make himself drink liquids when he was sick and his throat was sore, but it paid off in the long run.

Even without the Darth Vader mask, the infusion room nurse was always fun. He had a dry sense of humor and made all the patients laugh. His eyes were kind and he loved to give out warm blankets. Tom was feeling pretty good today, and they bantered as we walked down the hall.

I thought going into the infusion room would get easier over time, but it still made my stomach hurt. As we passed a mirror, I caught a glimpse of new wrinkles and whiter hair in my own reflection. I took a deep breath and focused on gratitude that this was the last infusion treatment.

All the nurses smiled and waved when Tom came into the room. I was sure he was one of their favorites. He was cooperative, didn't complain, and loved to share a story. He teased them when they wrapped the IV line in his arm with pink tape; he preferred the blue.

Part of my anxiety about the infusion room came from the seating. The patients were given oversized recliners that allow them to stretch out and rest during treatment. Getting the chairs to recline could sometimes be tricky, so the regulars help the newbies figure it out.

Tom looked so vulnerable in that chair.

I got him a warm blanket and worked it around the tubes coming out of his arm to get him covered. He got chilled easily those days. Bags of fluid hung from an IV pole that was to go wherever he went for the next eight hours. The room was full of people attached to similar poles.

Sometimes the infusion room made me think of musical chairs. While all the patient recliners had an IV pole beside them, they didn't all have a companion chair. Sometimes there weren't enough chairs for all the companions. Once I had to sit against a wall at his feet for the whole treatment, and another time I was temporarily parked in the hallway where I couldn't see him at all. That was hard.

But for this last one we had good seats. I sat beside him, and we talked all day. We always tried to talk about everything except why we were there—spiritual things; things to do at the Center; places we want to travel. I want to go to Europe—London and France. We both want to go to Alaska and see the Northern Lights. Usually the medications made him drowsy, and he napped. He was too excited to nap that day.

As his last bag of IV fluid started to get low, I saw the nurses preparing. I had been looking forward to this moment since our first day here.

Tom's ringing out ceremony.

All the nurses came to his chair, one of them ringing a bell. They cheered and congratulated him on his last chemo. They threw confetti all over him, gave him a glass of cranberry juice, placed beads around his neck, and gave him a certificate of completion signed by the whole staff.

Confetti got everywhere, and Tom doesn't care for cranberry juice, but he had a huge smile on his face.

We gathered all our stuff and headed for the door. He told the nurses he appreciated all they had done, but he never wanted to see them again. They said amen to that.

The elevator was packed with people as we left the building. It was a short quiet walk to the parking garage, and we got into the truck quickly. For a moment, all I could do was sit there with my hands on the steering wheel and breathe.

That was it. The last one.

"I couldn't have done it without you," Tom said quietly. We both had tears in our eyes as we pulled out of the parking lot and headed for home.

CHAPTER 30

Dawn was just beginning to break as I got out of bed. Sleep had been elusive, and I needed a shower to get me going. As I always do in these situations, I took a deep breath to calm my thoughts. It had been forty days since Tom's last appointment. I hadn't really counted until today, but there it was—forty days and forty nights. I probably should have felt the biblical significance of that number, but frankly, I was too tired.

Today Tom was to get a follow-up PET/CT scan, the first one since he finished his radiation treatments and chemotherapy. This one would tell us how well the treatments had worked.

I was glad to see that Tom looked better, felt better, and seemed more like his old self. But then he looked great, felt good, and was his old self before all this started. How quickly things can change.

I closed my eyes in the shower and used the water as a meditation aid. I visualized the water carrying away worry, negativity, and other energy I didn't need and wasn't helpful. The water was hot, and my body relaxed as my thoughts settled down.

Tom was sitting at the kitchen table with a glass of water when I came out of the bedroom. He took a sip and the look on his face left no doubt he would prefer his usual coffee. He was allowed to drink only water before the test.

A smile lit up his eyes when he saw me watching him. Even at his worst, there was still that light in his eyes when he smiled. Sometimes he was too sick to muster a smile, but when he did, it was better than the bank of stars shining on a clear desert night.

His appointment was early in the morning, and the promise of breakfast afterward was motivating enough to get us out the door ahead of schedule. We didn't talk much as he navigated rush hour traffic.

Since his scan was at the radiologist's office, it was an all too familiar route. We had done this drive every weekday for six weeks during his treatment. I had to remind myself to breathe as we got closer.

There was a parking spot available up front. Tom pulled in and turned off the truck, his hands lingering on the steering wheel as he let out a deep breath. I sat quietly to give him a moment. He looked over at me and I saw just a flash of uncertainty before it was replaced with a smile.

Nothing had changed in the waiting room. The same shows were on the television, something to do with buying houses or remodeling houses or tearing down houses or selling houses, houses being the operative theme. The energy in the room was still stifling and heavy with fear. The only thing that had changed were the patients sitting in the chairs. Different people with the same shell-shocked looks on their faces.

We found seats with a view of the TV, and I put my arm through his just to be close. Touching him soothed my nerves, though I knew that I should be soothing his. It never quite worked out that way.

The room was full and we waited just long enough to have an opinion about the house they were doing whatever they were doing to on the TV show before his name was called. I watched as he strode easily across the room and greeted the nurse with a friendly hello. He *was* almost like his old self again.

As he disappeared behind the door, my heart skipped a beat. He'd been through so much—we'd both been through so much. Enough was enough. It was time for this journey to end.

When he was finished, we were told we'd get the results in eight days. We got back in the truck and drove to breakfast. Now more than ever we knew that some things couldn't wait, that we should enjoy the good things each day had to bring, the simple things, like eating breakfast with the one you love.

Time seems to both drag and speed by when you are waiting for test results. Most tests have some amount of anxiety associated with them because they are, after all, tests. But waiting for health test results does especially weird things with time.

Tom's appointment was at 10:00 am. We had done the trip so many times that we have the drive time down perfectly and arrived the requested ten minutes early for the appointment. The waiting room was packed. We got the last two seats together and we were in luck because they faced the television.

I had to make an effort to keep my energy from getting jumpy. For my sake and everyone else's. There was enough uneasy energy in the room without me adding to it.

As usual the television was on HGTV. All the doctors' offices seem to show the same channel now. That's why we can't watch these shows at home; they remind us of these visits.

On a good day in the waiting room you don't get to see an entire show. Today it was Flea Market Flip, and it started soon after we arrived. In this half hour show, people buy junk, make it beautiful, and then sell it. Whoever does it best wins a prize. I've only watched it in waiting rooms, so I don't know all the nuances.

We watched a whole episode from start to finish.

Then another.

The doctor was running over an hour behind. I wanted him to hurry but at the same time I just wanted to sit there with Tom, watch TV and shut everything else out.

Finally, the nurse called him back to the room. She apologized for the wait while she took his vitals. He looked much better than the last time she saw him, and she told him that. The door closed behind her, and we sat quietly waiting for the doctor.

The doctor bustled in looking harried and apologizing for running behind, his assistant was out sick, and he was on his own today. He was quiet while he looked over Tom's test results.

Again, time seemed to go by instantly and take forever. In reality it was just a few moments before he looked up and said, "There is significant improvement."

I didn't know I had been holding my breath until I heard those words and started to breathe again. Tom looked over at me and smiled, the relief on his face evident.

Then the roller coaster went down the hill.

"It's not gone," the doctor said. "But the tumor is smaller, and the activity is down. There is some damage to the lung from radiation."

My head was swirling. Significant improvement should mean that everything was gone, and we could put this whole unpleasantness behind us. Why was the doctor still talking?

He told us about a new drug that had only had one study and was not yet FDA approved. It was not chemotherapy but immunotherapy. Immunotherapy works by stimulating the patient's immune system to recognize and destroy cancer cells. The drug is given intravenously every other week for a year. Unfortunately, it wasn't covered by insurance yet.

The look on Tom's face showed that he was as stunned as I was. If he had significant improvement, why did he need a drug that no one was sure would work?

"Without the drug, there is a 50% chance of recurrence. And if it does come back it will be Stage 4 and incurable," was the doctor's reply.

Then that also meant there was a 50% chance of NO recurrence.

There was some back and forth, but Tom said the drug just didn't feel right. The other option was to wait and do another scan. Standard protocol in this situation is to rescan in three months. Since the drug was very new on the scene, this seemed like a reasonable approach.

Tom decided to wait and rescan. He had been getting stronger every day and the doctor told us the chemo and radiation were both still working inside his body. We made a follow-up appointment and got copies of the results before leaving.

An elderly man entered the elevator ahead of us, and I felt Tom's hand tremble slightly as he guided me in next. The elevator stopped to pick up a woman on the second floor, when the doors opened I had a direct line of sight to the office where my mammograms are done. I worked hard to keep a check on my emotions. This building had so many memories.

We got to the bottom floor and headed out of the building. When we were finally alone on the sidewalk, Tom asked what I thought. I said a few unintelligible words, then burst into tears. I tried to explain that I wasn't crying because of the test results I was just overcome with the energy I had accumulated while we were in the office.

Crying vents the energy when I am overwhelmed. It's not pretty but it's effective.

I was actually hopeful from what I had heard. The doctor had said that supporting the immune system was the best course of action. He may only have one drug to offer, but as a trained naturopath I have other options.

When we got home, Tom asked me as many tough questions as he had asked the doctor. We made a plan and started implementing the easy things right away: lemon water; green smoothies; lots of vitamin C. He is no stranger to the dedication and hard work it takes to recover from a major health challenge.

We would do this.

CHAPTER 31

The door to my office flew open, and I jumped. When I looked up, Tom had a sheepish grin on his face and apologized for startling me. He headed through the office and into the house for lunch.

Even though Tom now regularly disrupted my work, I couldn't help but smile. It felt so good to have him well enough to burst through the door.

Tom had worked hard to recover from the chemotherapy and radiation treatments he received for lung cancer, and it was starting to show. He was back working in his studio turning wooden bowls and making custom art for his favorite clients. He was exercising regularly, and his wind capacity was better. He meditated and did bodywork to stay relaxed. He used castor oil packs and herbal remedies to improve his circulation and detoxify his body.

Slowly Tom was gaining back the weight he had lost during treatment. He was eating well and had even learned how to make green drinks in my Vitamix. These days, he was the one who made our afternoon smoothies.

Life was starting to seem normal again.

He poked his head around the corner and asked if I wanted to eat. A glance at the clock told me I had been sitting at my desk too long, so I decided it was a good time for a break. He offered to make egg burritos since the chickens had been laying fresh eggs again.

When my phone rang, the number looked familiar, so I answered. A voice I recognized as the assistant in the oncology office identified herself and asked how I was doing. We exchanged pleasantries, and then she got to the point.

The immunotherapy drug the oncologist had recommended at Tom's previous visit had been approved by the U.S. Food and Drug Administration (FDA). Just three days before, the drug had received fast track approval for treating Tom's type of lung cancer, and the treatment would be covered by insurance.

The doctor recommended this treatment for Tom. The sooner the better.

I caught my breath, thinking of all the pain and fear Tom had experienced during chemotherapy and radiation. The idea of him going through any part of that again made my heart hurt.

The nurse on the phone reminded me of the name of the drug and told me to look at the website. She said she would call back the next day. The doctor wanted a quick answer.

As I hung up the phone, I knew I needed to know more about immunotherapy. I did my research.

The immune system is a network of cells, tissues, and organs that work together to identify and destroy the body's foreign invaders— bacteria, viruses, parasites, fungus, and abnormal or unhealthy cells. The most important function of the immune system is to know the difference between the body's good tissue and the invaders.

Normally the immune system will not attack anything it recognizes as a healthy part of the body. Cancer cells are sneaky, however. They start out as regular cells the body recognizes as healthy, then they mutate, grow rapidly, and spread. Sometimes the immune system detects the changes and responds, but other times the cancer cells are able to outfox it. They hide from the immune system by using the cells' own immune on-off switch. If the switch is on, then the immune system doesn't attack the cancer cells.

The drug recommended for Tom is an immune checkpoint inhibitor. The immune system uses specific pathways to control the immune response to the foreign invaders. These pathways are called "immune checkpoints." These checkpoints hold the immune response in check so that healthy tissues are not damaged. Immune checkpoint inhibitors "inhibit"—that is, lessen—the ability of the checkpoints to hold back the immune response. In simpler terms, the drug turns the switch off so the immune system can target the cancer cells. These checkpoint inhibitors release the immune response, which in theory and as supported by clinical trials, then attacks and destroys the cancer cells that masquerade as healthy cells. One of the drawbacks, however, is that such a treatment can also attack and damage healthy cells.

I took all my research to Tom and told him what I knew about the drug, how it worked, and its possible side effects. The studies were promising, which is why it got fast tracked by the FDA. There are only a limited number of studies, however, and the long-term effects aren't known. The good news is that treatment with these kinds of drugs has more than tripled the length of time a patient can go without disease progression.

The most common side effects are fatigue, muscle aches, constipation, and nausea, but these aren't serious. The more serious side effects occur less often. With its brakes released, the immune system can go into overdrive and attack even the healthy parts of the body, such as the lungs, intestines, liver, hormone-making glands, kidneys, and other organs.

The dosing instructions were hard for Tom to hear—an IV-infusion every two weeks for a year. The procedure takes only an hour, but doing it for an entire year seemed daunting to both Tom and me. So much for pretending things were back to normal.

Since Tom needed to decide quickly, he talked with the oncologist by phone. His face remained neutral as he asked the doctor questions and listened to the answers. The doctor reminded Tom that he needed to start treatment right away. He was already past the recommended window after chemo to begin immunotherapy treatment.

Tom decided to sleep on it.

He got up the next morning and went about his normal routine. It was difficult for me to wait patiently, but I managed not to badger him with questions. After exercising, he went to his studio to work. It was lunch time when he came through the office door and sat down in the chair across from me.

"I'm going to do it," he said calmly. He had spent the morning meditating about this new treatment. Though not his first choice about how to spend time, he could spare an hour every two weeks, he decided, if it would hold off the progress of the disease three times as long as not doing the treatment. Those were odds he was willing to work with.

About three months later, Tom went in to receive the results of his CT scan. Eager to see how the immunotherapy was working, I went with him.

The doctor grinned when he entered the room. He shook our hands and looked at Tom. "How are you feeling?" he asked with a big smile.

"I feel great," Tom replied, and described some of the holistic approaches we were taking.

Clean eating	CBD and medical marijuana
Green drinks	Mindfulness and meditation
Energy medicine	Bodywork
Castor oil packs	Aromatherapy
Skin brushing	Herbal medicines

"That must be why you're doing so much better than many of my other patients," said the doctor, still grinning.

We stared at him in anticipation. We thought the news must be good, the way he was acting, but we wanted to hear it from him.

Well? Our faces were begging him to get on with it.

"Oh, right," the doctor said. "The scan looked good."

Talk about burying the lead. I felt my body relax. I didn't realize how tense I had been until that moment.

Relieved himself, Tom got chatty, telling the doctor he was back to his pre-diagnosis workout routine, and he could do everything he used to do. He admitted he got a little winded, though, when he worked too hard.

The doctor explained there was likely permanent damage to the lung from the radiation treatment. If Tom was getting "just a little winded," that was good news.

Tom's recovery was better than the norm and his doctor had noticed. He wanted to know more about the holistic therapies. He asked questions and seemed genuinely interested in the answers. Some of the therapies Tom used were recognizable to the doctor, but others required explanation.

Then Tom summed it up in one word, "Lifestyle. I've been on a holistic wellness journey for over 20 years, ever since Melanie started learning about herbs. Being healthy is important to me. I was in good health when I was diagnosed and during treatment I did as much as I could to keep up a healthy lifestyle. It was hard sometimes, but for every destructive thing that had to be done to eradicate the cancer, we balanced it with holistic therapy."

Tom looked at me and smiled. "I also have the most amazing woman by my side. She is more than just a loving, nurturing spirit. She knows holistic health. Having her there guiding me, and when necessary pushing me, through this journey made all the difference in the world."

I blushed at his compliment. His treatment and recovery had been a hard road and I was the most scared I had ever been in my life, but his words rang true. His determination and my knowledge had worked together for a positive outcome.

We make a hell of a team.

CONCLUSION

As you can tell, we are not at the end of our journey. I don't know yet how long it takes after you have cancer to rest easy. It has been two years since my diagnosis and surgeries. Apparently, it takes longer than that. My breast still hurts occasionally, usually when I haven't been tending to my own wellness.

When people ask me about cancer treatment this is what I tell them:

- Never make important decisions in the doctor's office.
- Who steps up to support you and who doesn't will surprise you.
- Focusing on your breath can help get you through anything.
- Stay present with your experiences.
- You know what is best for your body.
- Manage your pain, physical and emotional.
- It takes twice as long to heal as you plan for.

Tom is still undergoing immunotherapy treatment and will have CT scans every few months. His recovery has been nothing short of amazing. Just seven months after his last dose of chemo he is back to all the activities he did before the diagnosis. He works out regularly and is back to creating art in his shop. Even his hair, which he never lost completely, is returning to full strength.

I'd like to say that this experience has given us profound insights into the mysteries of the universe, but that's not quite the case. The insights we've gained have been small ones. How fragile is the nature of life. What hard, hard work it is to be ill, even in the 21st century.

That with education, persistence, and more than a little courage, you can take control of your own health and health care. That every day is a blessing. How very important it is to tell the ones you love that you love them, and as often as possible.

When you think about it, I guess these insights are pretty profound after all.

REFERENCES

Hay, Louise. Heal Your Body: The Mental Causes for Physical Illness and the Metaphysical Way to Overcome Them. Carlsbad, California: Hay House, 1984

Loeb, Lawrence A. "Human Cancers Express Mutator Phenotypes: Origin, Consequences and Targeting." Nature reviews. Cancer 11.6 (2011): 450–457. PMC. Web. 22 Aug. 2018.

https://www.webmd.com/cancer/pancoast-tumor#1

ABOUT MELANIE AND TOM DUNLAP

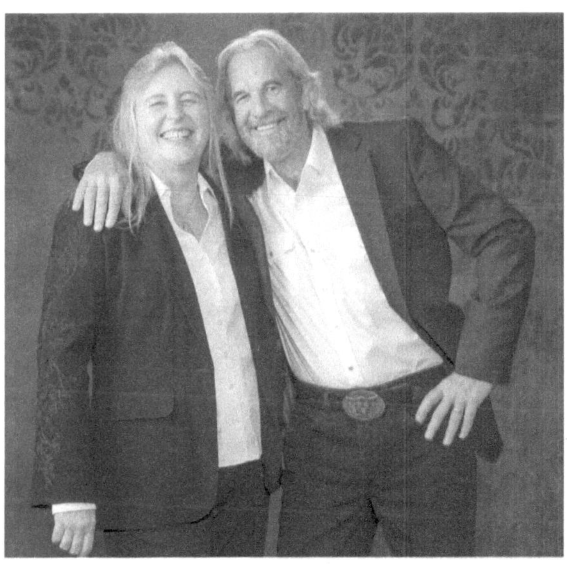

Married on a bet in 1984 (she won) the couple have traveled the United States, first in an 18-wheeler and later on a motorcycle. They have worked together most of their married life often being each other's boss. When not working for others they have been partners in entrepreneurial adventures. Most recently as co-founders of the Peaceful Spirit Enrichment Center in New River, AZ. www.PeacefulSpiritCenter.com

Tom is an award-winning artist and currently works in wood as a pyrographer. His art work is on display at the Peaceful Spirit Enrichment Center and the Hall of Flame Fire Truck Museum in Phoenix, AZ. www.ArtByDunlap.com

Melanie is a wise woman that loves plants, energy and natural healing. After decades of study in holistic health Melanie pursued a Doctor of Naturopathy degree from Trinity School of Natural Health. In her work as a wellness coach she combines her unique blend of intuition and knowledge to help women balance body, mind and spirit. www.MelanieDunlap.com